Coping with

with

LEUKEMIA

Melanie Ann Apel

The Rosen Publishing Group, Inc.
New York

616.994
APG

Published in 2001 by The Rosen Publishing Group, Inc.
29 East 21st Street, New York, NY 10010

Cover photo © Leif Skoogfors/CORBIS

Library of Congress Cataloging-in-Publication Data

Apel, Melanie Ann.
    Coping with leukemia / by Melanie Ann Apel.—1st ed.
        p.   cm.
    Includes bibliographical references and index.
    ISBN 0-8239-3200-1 (library binding)
    1. Leukemia—Juvenile literature. [1. Leukemia. 2. Diseases.]
I. Title.
    RC643 .A64   2000
    616.99'419—dc21   00-009847

Manufactured in the United States of America

About the Author

Melanie Ann Apel works as a pediatric respiratory therapist at Chicago's Children's Memorial Hospital. She holds
a bachelor of arts degree from Bradley University and
another from National-Louis University. When she is not
writing or taking care of sick children, Melanie loves figure skating and reading, and she is currently working on
learning how to relax. She has recently returned to her
native Chicago to be closer to her family.

Acknowledgments

The author wishes to extend thanks and love to Kathryn Beth Moskovitz for sharing her experiences with such honesty and to Mindy S. Apel for her detailed research assistance.

This book is dedicated to Kathryn Beth Moskovitz, who is winning her battle; to my dear and precious father, Darwin R. Apel, who has just begun his; and to the memories of my Uncle Larry Apel (1920–1994) and my dear Aunty Joy Moskovitz (1923–1999), whose fights were an inspiration to us all.

All my love, Melanie

Contents

Introduction   1

1 Leukemia   3

2 Symptoms   12

3 Diagnosis   17

4 Who Gets Leukemia and Why?   28

5 Chemotherapy   40

6 Radiation Therapy   50

7 Bone Marrow Transplants   58

8 Taking Care of Yourself   69

9 Living with Leukemia   78

10 Just for Teens   86

Glossary   97

Where to Go for Help   101

For Further Reading   102

Index   103

Introduction

Why did you pick up this book? Is it because you have just been diagnosed with leukemia? Is it because you have been in treatment for leukemia for some time and want to know more about your illness, or perhaps someone you know has leukemia or has just been diagnosed? Maybe you are just a curious person who likes to learn. Whatever your current health status, you have picked up this book, *Coping with Leukemia*, because you wish to learn more about leukemia and how to deal with it. In the pages that follow, various aspects of leukemia will be discussed, such as a description of symptoms, treatment options, and finally a list of books and resources that you can use to learn even more about this illness.

In the past, leukemia was considered terminal, meaning the diagnosed person would most likely die. Today, thanks to exhaustive research leading to major medical advances, many people who are diagnosed with leukemia can be treated and go on to live normal lives. It is truly amazing just how far medicine has come in terms of treating leukemia. There is a great deal of hope today. Whatever your reasons are for looking at this book, you are sure to learn a lot about leukemia and what you can do to cope if you, a friend, or a family member has been diagnosed.

Coping means meeting a challenge, facing adversity, holding up against the odds, and coming through it all in the end. Different people find different ways of coping with adverse situations. Some people are far better at coping when things go wrong than others are, but it is important to remember that the key to coping with an illness is understanding it. If you know what is happening to your body or if you can identify with what someone else may be going through, you will have a much easier time dealing with your feelings.

When you are done reading this book, you will understand what is going on inside the body of a person who has leukemia, you will know about the different types of leukemia, and you will have knowledge about treatment options. Finding out that you have an illness like leukemia can be very scary, but learning all you can about the illness can be your best tool for coping with your diagnosis. Reading this book is an excellent first step toward reaching your goal of coping with leukemia and, ultimately, having the strength and determination to fight the illness.

Leukemia

What is leukemia? Although this is a pretty straightforward question, there is no specific answer. Why not? Because leukemia is not one specific thing. The word "leukemia" is used to describe a group or collection of symptoms that have a particular effect on a person's body. The word "leukemia" actually means "white blood." Basically, leukemia is a form of cancer. Although you may have at one time or another heard someone say that leukemia is cancer of the blood, in fact it really is not. Although leukemia is not exactly "cancer of the blood," it is cancer of the cells and tissues that make blood. So you can see why people might make this mistake.

Leukemia is a condition in which a person's bone marrow—spongy red material that fills the center of the long and flat bones in your body—produces too many white blood cells too quickly. These extra cells are diseased and so they cannot do the things they would normally do in a healthy body, like fight off infections. As these extra white blood cells grow in number, they crowd out the red blood cells and the platelets. (You will read more about the blood and its components later in this chapter.) When all of these things start to go wrong in the bone marrow, a person has leukemia.

Because of the many badly functioning white blood cells and not enough red blood cells and platelets, a person who has leukemia will begin to feel sick. They will experience immense fatigue and easy bruising of the skin. Although leukemia affects children more often than adults, people can get leukemia at any age.

Leukemia is a complex disease and there are many different types, which is why there are many different treatment paths. The exact cause of leukemia is not really known, although there are several theories involving environment, heredity, and viruses. Before we get into specific discussions about the various aspects of leukemia, it is important for you to have some understanding of cancer in general.

What Is Cancer?

Just like leukemia itself, cancer is not one single disease. There are many different types of cancer When a person has cancer, the cells in his or her body are changing and growing in ways they are not supposed to. Instead of growing at their regular, steady rate, they grow wildly fast and out of control.

Most types of cancer involve tumors—a group of cancer cells that bunch together to form a mass or a lump. The lump can be very tiny or so big that it protrudes from the body and becomes visible from the outside. A tumor causes trouble when it blocks the passageways of systems within the body, such as blood flow. It can also press on an organ, keeping it from working to its full capacity, or cells from the tumor can break away from the original site

4

and start to travel around inside the body. When cancer cells travel to new areas of the body and grow there, metastasis has occurred. Cancer becomes more serious after it has begun to metastasize (muh-TAS-tuh-size).

An interesting point about metastatic cancer is that even if the cancer has metastasized to another part of the body, it keeps the name of its original site. This is sort of like if you were born in America and move to Ireland, you are still considered to be an American. The same holds true for metastatic cancer because if the cancer originates in the bones and then moves to the lungs, it is still considered bone cancer, not lung cancer.

Another word for cancer, which you may have heard is "malignancy." When a person is diagnosed with a tumor, the doctors must find out whether the tumor is malignant or benign (which means not cancerous). Although a cancerous, or malignant, tumor is usually more serious than a benign tumor, a benign tumor can also cause serious problems in the body, depending on where it is, what it is pressing against, and what body systems it is interfering with. However, what makes a tumor benign is the fact that it does not grow or spread around the body the way a malignant tumor does. But not all cancers form tumors. In fact, leukemia does not form tumors.

Is Leukemia Cancer?

Yes, leukemia is a form of cancer. Many people get cancer and many people survive cancer. You probably have heard people say they wish there was one cure for all

5

cancers. This will probably never happen, even though there are some curable forms of cancer already, and eventually all forms of cancer may be curable. But chances are each type of cancer will have its very own cure, just as various forms of cancer right now have their own types of treatment and different prognoses, or prospects of recovery. There will most likely never be one "all purpose" cure for cancer.

Let us now take a look at leukemia as cancer. Leukemia is cancer of the white blood cells, which are a part of what makes up our blood. It starts in the bone marrow, which is made of cells that form blood, fat cells, and tissues that help the blood cells grow. If you have a dog, you may feed him or her dog treats that are made to look like slices of bone. Typically they consist of a white ring (the bone part) filled with a red substance, which represents the bone marrow. It is here, inside the bone marrow, that all of the different types of blood cells are manufactured. When you were a baby, almost all of your bones were filled with bone marrow. Now that you are a teenager, however, you store most of your bone marrow in your flat bones, which are the skull, ribs, backbone, pelvis, and shoulder blades.

Leukemia spreads from the bone marrow out to the blood, lymph nodes, spleen, liver, central nervous system, and then to other organs in the body. Aside from the fact that leukemia does not form tumors, leukemia is also different from other cancers in that it starts in the bone marrow and spreads through the body. Other cancers start in an organ and spread through the body, sometimes making their way to the bone marrow.

Blood and Blood Cells

You are certainly familiar with your own blood, as you have probably cut yourself on many occasions. But aside from the fact that your blood is red, what else do you know about it?

Blood is one of the most important liquids inside your body. You can think of it as being a messenger service, dropping off important products where they need to go and then picking up the waste afterward. Blood carries oxygen, vital nutrients, hormones, food, and all the other things your body needs to satisfy its tissues and cells. It also picks up the toxins and waste products from the cells and gets rid of them. Blood helps your body fight infection by working with the lymph system (which will be discussed later in this chapter). It also delivers the cells that your body needs to repair injuries, such as when you cut yourself. Vital clotting factors, which keep your body from bleeding uncontrollably when you are injured, are also the responsibility of the blood. So as you can see, blood performs several functions that keep people alive.

Blood is made up of several components. Whole blood, which is the blood you see when you cut yourself, is made of clear fluid called plasma and a team of other things, each doing a specific job. Only three of these blood components are really involved in leukemia: white blood cells, red blood cells, and platelets.

In order to understand what goes wrong inside the body of a person who has leukemia, it will help if you understand something about blood and blood cells. In addition to bone marrow, the blood system involves red blood cells, white blood cells, platelets, and the lymphatic system. Each component of the blood has a very specific job to do. If one or more of these components cannot function properly, there will be big problems inside the body. Young blood cells are called primitive blood cells or stem cells, and as these stem cells grow and mature in an orderly manner, they produce red blood cells, white blood cells, and platelets.

Red Blood Cells
The job of the red blood cells, also known as erythrocytes, is to carry oxygen away from the lungs and out to all of the other systems and tissues in the body. A protein in the red blood cells, called hemoglobin, is responsible for making blood red and for oxygen transport. You can think of hemoglobin as the bus that the oxygen rides to get where it is going. After the red blood cells deliver the oxygen, they pick up the waste product of all cell activity, namely carbon dioxide. If the body runs short of red blood cells, a person is said to be suffering from a condition called anemia. Symptoms of anemia include weakness and tiredness, as well as shortness of breath. Usually a person can take iron pills or eat iron-rich foods to build up his or her supply of red blood cells.

Platelets
Platelets, also known as thrombocytes, are pieces that have broken off from some of the bone marrow cells. The reason they are called platelets is because when you look at them under a microscope, you will notice that they resemble small plates or discs. The job of platelets is to

help prevent excess bleeding in your body by plugging up places on the blood vessels that have become damaged, like if you cut or bruise yourself. If you have ever had a scab form over a cut on your body, then you have seen firsthand your platelets at work. Leukemia slows down the rate at which platelets are made. This is why people who have leukemia may experience frequent nosebleeds, gum bleeds, and chronic bruising.

White Blood Cells

White blood cells are also called leukocytes. Look carefully at the prefix *leuk-*. The *leuk-* is the same prefix as in the word "leukemia," which tells you that leukemia has something to do with white blood cells, which you already know. The suffix *–cyte* means cell. The job of the white blood cells is to help the body defend itself against infections that are caused by germs, such as bacteria, viruses, and fungi. White blood cells hang out in the bone marrow until they are needed to fight germs. When your body has an infection, your bone marrow makes more white blood cells to help out in the battle to get rid of the infection. There are two main types of white blood cells. These are granulocytes and lymphocytes. Each plays a very specific role in protecting your body from infection. There are four types of granulocytes that step up for the fight when your body has an infection that is making you sick.

- Basophils are the rarest of all white blood cells. Their job is to protect you from allergic reactions.

- Eosinophils help fight off parasites and bad bacteria. They also respond to allergic reactions.

 Monocytes have special enzymes that kill off bad bacteria.

 Neutrophils are the largest group of white blood cells. They are also responsible for destroying bad bacteria.

You may wonder why the word "bad" has been used to describe bacteria. Did you think that all bacteria were bad? In fact, your body is filled with good bacteria that it needs to keep a healthy balance inside. It is when foreign or bad bacteria get into your body and upset the balance that you get sick.

There are two kinds of lymphocytes, and their job is to prevent infection before it has a chance to get into your body and make you sick. T cells are cells that attack cancer cells, infected cells, and foreign bodies such as transplanted organs. You will hear a great deal about T cells when you have leukemia. B cells, on the other hand, are responsible for making antibodies to kill off foreign substances that find their way into your body. Overall, each kind of leukemia has to do with one of the types of white blood cells being cancerous.

The Lymphatic System

The lymphatic system is a complex system that resembles the veins but carries a substance other than blood. Lymph nodes, lymph vessels, and lymph fluid make up the lymphatic system. The lymph vessels resemble the veins in the body. However, instead of carrying blood through the body, they carry lymph fluid—a clear liquid made up of the extra fluid from the tissues in the body, waste products, and immune system cells. Lymph nodes, which are also often referred to as lymph glands, are actually organs. They are very small, about the size of a pea, and they are found running along the lymph vessels. The job of the lymph nodes is to collect immune system cells.

When your body is fighting an infection, you may notice that your lymph nodes are swollen. Your doctor will check for this by gently running his or her hands under your jaw and up and down the sides of your neck. You also have lymph nodes under your armpits and in your groin area. Although swollen lymph nodes are not by themselves a problem, they do sometimes indicate a problem inside the body such as mononucleosis or leukemia.

Now that you have some understanding of what the blood and lymph systems do inside the body, you are ready to learn more about leukemia.

Symptoms

If you have leukemia, you may have been sick for a while and not known what was wrong with you before you were finally diagnosed. This happens sometimes because the symptoms of leukemia are rather vague and are also similar to many common illnesses, such as the flu. Your first symptom of leukemia was probably a familiar and general feeling of being run-down.

Recognizable Symptoms

If you are not a person who has been diagnosed with leukemia, keep in mind that even if you have several of the following symptoms, you do not necessarily have leukemia. You could have any number of other illnesses or no illness at all. Only a doctor can tell you for sure whether or not you actually have leukemia, so do not panic if some of the symptoms sound familiar to you. In general, symptoms of leukemia can include:

- Fatigue and weakness

- Loss of weight

- Fever

- Decrease or loss of appetite

- Anemia

- Shortness of breath

- Pale skin

- Chronic bruising

- Bleeding gums and frequent, severe nosebleeds

- Headaches

- Seizures

- Vomiting

- Problems keeping your balance

- Blurry vision

- Pain in your bones and joints

- Swelling of the liver, spleen, or joints

- Skin rash

- Coughing

Chances are, even if you have been diagnosed with leukemia, you had only some of these symptoms. One of the reasons for this is that not all types of leukemia produce the same set of symptoms. Let's look at a breakdown of why a person who has leukemia might experience some, but not all, of the symptoms mentioned in the list above.

The majority of symptoms that indicate a person has acute leukemia are due to a shortage of normal blood cells in the body. This shortage is a result of the leukemia cells crowding out the bone marrow cells that produce healthy blood cells. The leukemia cells take over, making it difficult for the body to make and store enough red blood cells, white blood cells, and platelets to keep the body healthy, running properly, and feeling good. However, these symptoms could be caused by so many other things that it is easy to see how a diagnosis of leukemia may be missed at first.

The first five symptoms on the list—fatigue, weakness, loss of weight, fever, and decrease or loss of appetite—are the most common symptoms and probably the first to appear when leukemia starts to affect a person's body. Headaches, seizures, vomiting, balance problems, and blurry vision are symptoms that show the leukemia has made its way out of the bone marrow and has invaded the body's other organs, as well as the central nervous system. Joint pain and bone pain occur when leukemia cells spread from the bone marrow out to the surface of the joints and bones. If the leukemia cells make their way to the liver, the spleen, or the lymph nodes, these organs will swell.

People who have a certain type of leukemia called acute myelogenous leukemia may experience some swelling in their mouth, because this type of leukemia spreads into the gums, making them bleed. If a skin rash develops, it may be because the acute myelogenous leukemia cells have also spread to the skin.

Involvement of the Thymus and Superior Vena Cava

The thymus is a ductless, glandlike organ in the upper chest near the throat. The function of the thymus is not known, although T cell–type acute lymphocytic leukemia frequently involves the thymus. Inside your body there is a very large vein that carries blood from your head and arms back to your heart. This vein is called the superior vena cava and it runs right by the thymus. If the leukemia has gotten into the thymus and made it larger, the swollen thymus can cause problems for the superior vena cava by pressing on it. The thymus will then also press on the trachea (your windpipe), making you cough and feel short of breath. The worst case scenario is that pressure on the trachea could actually close it off, causing a person to suffocate and die. Another problem that can happen if the leukemia cells get in the way of the superior vena cava is that the compression can cause the head and arms to swell. This is very dangerous, even life threatening. In fact, this condition is so serious that it has its very own name: SVC syndrome. A person suffering from SVC syndrome needs immediate medical attention and care.

Anemia

Anemia is a specific condition that occurs when a person's body is not able to make enough red blood cells. When a person has anemia, he or she is said to be anemic. People who do not have leukemia can become anemic for different reasons, so it is important to understand that just because a person has anemia does not automatically mean that she or he also has leukemia.

Anemia causes a variety of general symptoms, such as shortness of breath, tiredness, and pale skin. The first two of these symptoms can have many causes other than anemia. You can probably think of a lot of different reasons for being tired. Shortness of breath can be caused by exercise, asthma, or smoking. So it is the paleness of the skin that is the biggest indicator of a problem. But keep in mind, you may be pale for other reasons. Perhaps it is winter and you have not been out in the sunshine for months or you might have the flu. Pale skin does not always mean a person has anemia or leukemia. However, if these three symptoms all show up, then your best bet is to pay a visit to your doctor and see what is going on. If you have anemia, there are simple things you can do to recover. Your doctor may prescribe iron tablets or advise you to change your diet to include more foods that are rich in iron, like spinach and liver. If your anemia is a symptom of a more serious illness, namely leukemia, you will need to start more aggressive treatment right away. Treatment for leukemia will be discussed in detail later on in this book in chapters 5 and 6.

It is important to remember that many of the symptoms of leukemia can also be symptoms of something else, like another serious illness, or nothing at all. Only your doctor can tell you for certain why you are experiencing your symptoms. Do not just panic and assume that you have leukemia. If you are worried, you can set your mind at ease by seeing a doctor. Then if your symptoms do turn out to be leukemia, it will be advantageous that you caught it early and can get the treatment you need to get well.

Diagnosis

Even though doctors and scientists have been researching what makes a person get leukemia, they still do not know the exact cause. They have made a great deal of progress in this area, and they will continue to work until they know the reasons so many people are plagued by cancers like leukemia.

Ian has not been feeling like himself lately. Usually in the afternoons he loves to get a basketball game going in the park by his house. He plays with Chris and Cordell and sometimes his little brother TJ joins in. They play until it's dark out and someone's mom or dad calls the boys in for dinner. But for the past few weeks Ian has been so exhausted after school that all he wants to do is take a nap until dinnertime.

"What's the matter with you?" Cordell asks him one afternoon.

"I don't know."

"You sleep as much as my baby sister," Chris says.

"Well, I'm tired."

"Maybe you have mono," says Cordell "My sister Lilly had that when she was a senior."

"I'm not sick, I'm just tired. Let's play ball," Ian says, annoyed at being compared to a baby and accused of being sick. Ian picks up the ball and

shoots at the basket. He and his friends play for a few minutes, but soon Ian is so tired he is stumbling. Chris bumps into him in an attempt to get the ball from him, and Ian falls down on the court. It is not long before a large bruise starts to form on Ian's leg.

"Hey, sorry, man," Chris says.

"No problem," Ian says and picks up the ball again.

"Ian!" Cordell shouts, before Ian even has a chance to make another basket. "Your nose is bleeding!"

Blood is all over the place. Chris runs across the street to get Ian's mom and dad while Cordell sits on the court with Ian.

"What's wrong with me?" Ian whispers.

Your doctor will do several things when he or she is trying to figure out what is making you sick. The first thing he or she will do is inquire about your history or background. All this means is that your doctor or a nurse will ask you or your parents a series of questions about your recent health, activities, vacations, and social life. You may be asked if you have experienced any of the symptoms of leukemia. Certain types of leukemia cause other symptoms, so your doctor may also ask you if you have had night sweats, irritability, or infections that do not respond to medication. Then your doctor will examine you, looking for such things as bruises, enlarged lymph nodes, an enlarged liver, and an enlarged spleen. The doctor may also look under your hair for a pale green mark, indicating a chloroma—a tumor, which is a symptom of acute myelogenous leukemia.

Next, your doctor will take a sample of your blood to look for a low red blood cell count, a low platelet count, either an especially high or an especially low white blood cell count, and blast cells—mature blood cells that do not grow and age normally. Having blood drawn may sound scary but here is an easy trick you can use if you are worried about the needle. If needles bother you, tell your doctor that you do not want to see it. Hold your arm steady and either close your eyes or look away.

If your doctor still suspects that you have leukemia after the questions, exam, and blood test, you will have to have your bone marrow tested. A sample of your bone marrow is drawn from your spine or your hip using a very large needle. This procedure can be painful, but your doctor will give you medication that will numb the area where the needle will be inserted so that you will not feel the puncture. You may be a bit sore for a day or so after this procedure.

Your doctor will then send your bone marrow sample on to a pediatric oncologist, a doctor who specializes in children's cancer, or a pathologist, a doctor who specializes in analyzing body tissues. The pathologist will look at your tissue sample under a microscope to determine whether or not you actually have leukemia. If this doctor finds that your bone marrow is made up of more than 25 percent blasts, leukemia is diagnosed.

Your bone marrow is then sent to another laboratory where the leukemia cells are analyzed to figure out which kind of leukemia you have. Different kinds of leukemia respond to different types of treatment, so it is important to know which kind of leukemia you have.

Every once in a while, children and teens are diagnosed with leukemia when they are not even feeling sick.

Although this sounds frightening, finding out that you have leukemia before you show symptoms is advantageous because it means that the leukemia has not advanced very far. Most likely, the leukemia is still in very early stages, making the prognosis even more promising.

"I was just going for my yearly doctor visit. I think it may have been the one I had to go to before I went to junior high school," says David, now almost sixteen. "I felt fine. It was the middle of August and I had spent all summer on the beach with my cousins. I was tan and I felt healthy. No one would ever have guessed that I was sick. Even I had no idea. When I went to the doctor for the checkup, she took blood for a regular blood test. It was just a routine thing, like she always did.

A few days later my doctor called and told my mom to bring me over to the office right away. My mom and I drove right over and we could tell that my doctor had some bad news because she had a sort of worried look on her face.

She told me that my blood test had come back and that there was a problem. She was pretty sure that I had leukemia. I was shocked because I still felt fine, although I had started to feel a little bit tired during the week right before. I thought I was just staying outside too long in the evenings or something. My mom got really upset and started to cry.

My doctor said that she would have to do some more tests on me. So I had a few more blood tests and a bone marrow test. Sure enough, the tests all came back positive and I had leukemia. Luckily though, since my doctor caught it so early, I was doing really great by Christmas that year. I was already in remission. It was pretty cool. I hardly even remember being sick. It was such a short period of time. I got well really fast."

Important Terms

Leukemia actually refers to several different illnesses that are related to cancer and white blood cells. Before we start our discussion about the various types of leukemia, you will need to be familiar with the following terms.

Acute

This term generally means "sudden onset." In other words, the leukemia develops quickly. In leukemia that is considered acute, white blood cells grow too quickly, leaving them unable to mature properly and therefore unable to perform their proper function. Leukemia is identified as acute if there is an abnormal—too high or too low—number of immature white blood cells. Most children and teens who have leukemia have an acute form.

Chronic

Chronic means long-term, and chronic leukemia develops slowly. In chronic leukemia, white blood cells look as if they have had a chance to mature, but in fact they have not and so they are considered abnormal cells. They live longer than they are supposed to, building up and causing problems in the body. Only 5 percent of all cases of leukemia in children are chronic.

Lymphocytic and Myelogenous
Lymphocytic leukemia stems from lymphocytes in the bone marrow. In contrast, myelogenous, sometimes called myeloid or myelocytic, begins from one of two types of white blood cells, the monocytes or the granu-loycytes. Each type of leukemia is either acute or chronic and lymphocytic or myelogenous.

Types of Leukemia in Children

There are four types of leukemia, and both children and adults can get any type. However, certain types of leukemia are found more often in specific age groups.

- ✑ Acute lymphocytic leukemia (ALL) accounts for just over half of all cases of childhood leukemia. This type affects both children and adults.

- ✑ Chronic lymphocytic leukemia (CLL) affects adults and is almost twice as common as chronic myelogenous leukemia.

- ✑ Acute myelogenous leukemia (AML) affects both children and adults and accounts for just under half of all cases of childhood leukemia.

- ✑ Chronic myelogenous leukemia (CML) is very rare in children and in adults is about half as common as chronic lymphocytic leukemia.

Acute Lymphocytic Leukemia
Most children who have leukemia have acute lymphocytic leukemia (ALL). Acute lymphocytic leukemia happens as a

result of a genetic injury to the DNA of a single cell in the bone marrow. It is not a hereditary injury. It is something that happens to the person who gets sick.

If you have acute lymphocytic leukemia, two main things are happening to your blood. The first is that there is an uncontrolled growth of cells called lymphoblasts or leukemic blasts. These blast cells do not function the way normal blood cells do. The other thing that is happening is that normal bone marrow cells are not able to form, leaving your body without enough red blood cells, platelets, and normal white blood cells. Scientists have not had an easy time pinpointing the exact cause of acute lymphocytic leukemia, although exposure to high doses of radiation has been associated with its origination.

What scientists have discovered is that acute lymphocytic leukemia occurs at different rates in different areas of the country. They have also discovered that there are higher rates of leukemia in developed countries than in underdeveloped countries. But they are not sure why this is true. One suspicion is that leukemia may be caused by exposure to infection or toxic agents during fetal development or as a very young child. Acute lymphocytic leukemia is most often seen in children under ten years old and in much older adults, with the greatest risk being in the first five years of a child's life.

Acute Myelogenous Leukemia

Acute myelogenous leukemia (AML), also called acute non-lymphocytic leukemia or acute myelogenoid leukemia, is less common than acute lymphocytic leukemia and has several subtypes. One characteristic of acute myelogenous leukemia is that children who have Down's syndrome have a greater risk than other children of developing AML during the first three years of their life. In rare cases of acute myelogenous leukemia, tumor cells appear. A solid tumor that develops is called an isolated granulocytic sarcoma or chloroma.

Both children and adults can get acute myelogenous leukemia. Your doctor will have to look at the chromosomes of your leukemia cells to decide whether you have AML or ALL. By the time acute myelogenous leukemia is diagnosed, it will have already spread through your bloodstream. The main way of treating acute myelogenous leukemia is with chemotherapy, and if this is not effective, a bone marrow transplant may become necessary. Sometimes, but not often, radiation is also used to treat acute myelogenous leukemia if you have developed a tumor.

Tess sits in the exam room of her doctor's office, watching her mom pretend to read a book. Tess can tell that her mother is nervous. She keeps glancing around the room. Tess is nervous, too.

It has been only two weeks since she came to see the doctor for her yearly checkup, and Dr. Ottenfeld had told her that everything was fine. She was growing well and appeared to be quite healthy. But the week after she saw Dr. Ottenfeld, Tess started to have fevers. She was very tired and felt terribly weak. School was about to start, but she could not imagine having the energy to go. Tess's mother guessed that she just had a bad case of the flu.

Tess's mom called Dr. Ottenfeld, and he said to bring her in to the office right away. Dr. Ottenfeld took blood from Tess's arm and then sent her home to rest. Last night, Dr. Ottenfeld called and told her mom to bring her in again this morning.

"Is it bad news?" Tess blurts out the moment Dr. Ottenfeld walks into the exam room where she and her mom are waiting. "Is something wrong with me?"

Dr. Ottenfeld appears concerned as he looks at Tess's pale face and notices that she has lost a bit of weight since she was in the office just two weeks ago.

"Well, Tess, your preliminary blood work indicates that you have leukemia," Dr. Ottenfeld says gently.

"But why? How did I get this?" Tess asks, confused. "I was fine two weeks ago."

"I know you were," Dr. Ottenfeld agrees. "We really do not know why people get leukemia."

Finding Out

Everyone reacts differently when they first hear they have leukemia. You may have been shocked, scared, or worried. You may have been in denial and thought that your doctor was lying to you. You may have been very quiet, needing to digest the information, or you may have screamed and cried. You may not have told anyone right away or you may have told everyone you know. You are the one who has leukemia, and your reaction is very much your own. No one can tell you how you should react or how you should feel.

It is very important to deal with your feelings. Experience them. Understand and go through your emotions. When you are able to deal with your feelings about leukemia, you will be able to begin your fight against it.

Friends, Family, and Your Reaction

How you react to your diagnosis of leukemia is a very personal thing. While some people may be very angry and sad, others may accept their diagnosis and want to get started on treatment right away. There is no wrong reaction to finding out that you have leukemia. In most cases, your emotions will dictate your actions. No one can deny that finding out that you have leukemia is frightening and upsetting. Feelings that you may have experienced when you first learned of your leukemia include fear, anger, denial, depression, sadness, and hopelessness.

You may have noticed that you were not the only person in your family to have one or more of these reactions. Certainly your mom and dad may have been just as upset as you were when they found out that you have leukemia. If you have brothers and sisters, they may have had reactions of their own as well. Close family members and friends may also be upset by your diagnosis. It is okay for other people to be upset, even though you are the only one who is actually sick. They care about you and want you to be well. Share your feelings with those people who are close to you and encourage them to share their feelings about your illness with you.

"When I first got sick," says Ivan, fourteen, "I was afraid to talk to anyone in my family about it. I thought it would upset them if they knew how scared I felt. My little brother Nic, who was only eight, started acting really strange. He hardly talked to me at all. I finally had to ask him what was up and when

I did he started crying and saying that he was afraid that I was going to die. Well, I assured him that I was going to do everything I could to get better so that we could grow up together.

"Nic felt a lot better after we talked and he started acting like his old normal self again. But the weirdest part was that I felt better, too. I realized that we were all afraid of what might happen to me, and that talking about it really made us all feel better. Now I let Nic know exactly what is going on with me and my treatments and stuff, and he asks me lots of questions."

If you do not understand what is going on inside your body when you have leukemia, it is natural for you to be frightened by the way your body feels. Knowing what is happening and what the doctors and are going to do to help you fight the leukemia will help make the unknown more understandable. You will not feel as afraid. Talking to your nurses and doctors, asking them to answer any and all questions you may have will help set you at ease. Remember, this is your body and your life, and therefore you have the right to know what is going on. You can be part of your own Get Well Team. After all, you are the one who has to fight the hardest for your health. It helps to understand exactly what is being done for you and how your body might react to the various treatments.

Who Gets Leukemia and Why?

Leukemia has been around for a very long time. The first time that doctors observed and wrote about a condition in which patients had great elevations in their white blood cell count was in nineteenth-century Europe. The term "weiss blut," meaning "white blood" was the name they gave to this disorder, and the name leukemia came later.

When you hear the word "leukemia," you most likely think of a sick child, but as you now know, anyone can get leukemia at any age. One thing to keep in mind, however, is that some people are more likely than others to get leukemia. Likewise, some people are more likely to be successfully treated for their leukemia than others. Of course, this is not to say that if you fall into a certain category that you definitely will get leukemia, or that you will not be successfully treated if you do get it. In addition to the treatments prescribed by your doctor, your best defense against leukemia is a good attitude and a positive outlook.

Statistics

Of all the kinds of cancer that people can get, acute leukemia is the one that is the most common in children.

But actually, as you can see from the statistics below, more adults than children get this kind of cancer.

- Approximately 2,500 children are diagnosed with acute leukemia every year in the United States.

- Approximately 25,000 adults are diagnosed with acute leukemia every year in the United States.

- Childhood leukemia is usually diagnosed between the ages of two and seven.

- The highest incidence of childhood leukemia is in children who are four years old.

- Leukemia is more common in Caucasians than in African Americans.

- More boys than girls get leukemia.

- Children who already have a genetic disease such as Down's syndrome or Fanconi's anemia have a higher risk for developing leukemia.

- The number of children who get cancer every year has been increasing steadily for the past thirty years.

- Most children who have leukemia have an acute form.

- Only 5 percent of children who have leukemia have a chronic form.

Heredity

Researchers do not know if leukemia is an inherited disease. They have been able to figure out that the deoxyribonucleic acid (DNA), the chemical responsible for carrying instructions to all of the cells in your body, changes when a person has leukemia. These changes seem to happen after a person is born, rather than before. But why do these DNA mutations happen? This is a very good question. Researchers have been trying to answer this question for years, and it is only recently that they have learned that certain changes in a person's DNA can make the cells in the bone marrow develop into leukemia.

DNA, Genes, and Oncogenes

DNA controls how things are put together both on the inside of your body and the outside of your body. For example, DNA passed on to you from your mom and dad is what makes you look like your parents. You have probably heard of genes. They are the part of DNA that contains the actual instructions that tell your body's cells when to grow and divide normally. Oncogenes, on the other hand, are the specific genes responsible for this cell division. Tumor suppressor genes are responsible for slowing down cell growth and division and making sure that cells die off.

When a person gets cancer, mutations in the DNA can cause one of two things to happen. Either the oncogenes turn on, making the cells grow and divide out of control, or the tumor suppressor genes turn off, which also causes the cells to grow and act abnormally.

Another problem that can occur happens during the time a cell is getting ready to divide into two new cells and it is supposed to make a copy of its DNA. Because the process is not a perfect one, sometimes there is a problem in the copying process. Think of it this way: Usually when you are using a photocopy machine, it works just fine and you get all the copies you need, but sometimes there is a glitch. A problem might occur that has to be fixed, such as a paper jam caused by too many sheets of paper going through at once. Sometimes you can correct this on your own, but other times a repairman may need to be called to fix the copier. Likewise, most of the time even if the cell makes a mistake when it is copying its DNA there is a special enzyme in the cell that proofreads the DNA and corrects any errors before they can cause any serious damage. However, if a cell starts to grow and divide too quickly, the repair enzymes may not be able to catch all of the errors and some may slip by and start to cause problems.

Translocation

Another DNA problem that can lead to leukemia is called translocation. Translocation is when DNA from one chromosome attaches itself to the wrong chromosome after division. This is a mistake that can cause the oncogenes to come in and start to work overtime. Translocation of different chromosomes is responsible for different types of leukemia. Doctors can test to see if this is the cause of a person's leukemia. The results of such a test can help discover whether or not a person actually has leukemia and what the prognosis is for that person, and it can also be used to see if leukemia has come back following treatment.

Environmental Influences

Changes in DNA that create leukemia can be caused by several environmental factors. Among the most common are radiation and chemical exposures. When people have accidentally or sometimes intentionally been exposed to radiation or carcinogens—specific cancer-causing chemicals—their risk for developing leukemia may increase.

Chemical Spills

You may have heard about a place called Hiroshima. This was a town in Japan that was hit by an atomic bomb during World War II. Many people died right after the bomb hit, but many others who initially survived the bombing got sick later. In the years following the bombing, these people developed leukemia and other forms of cancer because they had been exposed to strong doses of radiation and chemicals. This was, of course, an extreme case of radiation poisoning.

Another example of a large dose of radiation that you may have read about in your history class was the Chernobyl accident in the Ukraine. Chernobyl, as you may know, was the site of the world's worst nuclear power accident. In April 1986, the Chernobyl nuclear power plant was testing one of its four nuclear reactors when a chain reaction in the reactor got out of control. The result was an explosion with a fireball so big that it blew off the reactor's steel and concrete lid. The accident at Chernobyl killed more than thirty people right away, but the excessively high radiation levels spread out over a surrounding twenty-mile radius, causing 135,000 people to be evacuated from their homes. Since the Chernobyl accident, the cancer rate in Ukrainian children, from birth to fifteen years old, has risen from four to six incidents per million to forty-five incidents per million.

Home and Job-Related Exposure

Depending on what kind of job they have, some adults are exposed to small amounts of radiation over a long period of time. Eventually this radiation exposure begins to affect the insides of their bodies, and they develop leukemia or other forms of cancer.

In recent years, environmentalists have also become very concerned about certain areas of the country in which the number of people who have developed leukemia seems much higher than in other areas. Contaminated water supplies, power lines, garbage dumps, certain building materials, and other environmentally hazardous entities are thought to be responsible for increased risks of cancers in certain populations. Environmental problems aside, DNA mutations can also happen for no known reason.

Down Syndrome and Genetic Diseases

Children who have genetic diseases such as Down syndrome have an extra chromosome. What this means is that they have more genetic material in their cells than they are supposed to have or that they have abnormal chromosomes. These abnormalities lead to a higher chance of developing leukemia, but experts do not really know whether they actually cause the leukemia or if it just happens that the two problems often occur together.

One reason why it is thought that there is possibly a genetic link to developing leukemia is that if one identical twin gets leukemia, there is a 25 percent chance that his or her twin will also get leukemia. However, the older the children get, the lower that risk becomes. Of course, this increase in risk could be a result of environment rather than heredity, since twins are usually raised together and are therefore exposed to the same environmental factors or carcinogens. Once again, there is really no definite answer as to whether leukemia is hereditary or caused by environmental factors.

Could It Be a Virus?

If you have ever been sick with a cold or the flu, you have had a virus in your body. It is not unusual for people to pick up viruses that make them sick, especially in the winter. In fact, it is so common for people to get sick with a cold virus that the cold is often referred to as "the common cold." Viruses are tricky little germs. They cannot be killed by most medication, which is why there is no cure for a cold or the flu. Sure, you can take medicines to relieve some of your symptoms, but your cold or flu will stick around until it has run its course.

Sometimes colds and flus leave behind damage even after the original sickness has left the body. Scientists wondered if perhaps this is how people get leukemia. Research has found that mice, cats, cows, chickens, and a monkey called the gibbon all get leukemia when they are exposed to a certain virus.

It has also been found that lymphoma, a very rare kind of leukemia that adults occasionally get, is caused by a T cell virus. However, researchers still cannot find any virus that is responsible for the types of leukemia that children can get. So the answer is no, it does not appear to be viruses that cause most types of leukemia.

So What Is the Cause?

You have learned that leukemia is not contagious, not specifically genetic, not caused by any known specific virus, and that most children who get leukemia are not old enough to have been exposed to large doses of radiation or chemicals. So what causes a person to get leukemia? No one knows for certain.

Currently, experts believe a complex interaction involving all of the above factors—environment, heredity, the immune system, and perhaps something viral—causes some people, but not others, to develop leukemia. As it is very unlikely for more than one person in a family to develop leukemia, it is pretty easy to say that there is nothing anyone can do to predict who is going to get leukemia and who is not. So it is safe to say, in other words, that it is never anyone's fault when someone gets leukemia.

Can Leukemia Be Prevented?

Since a specific cause for leukemia has not yet been identified, it is unfortunately true that at this time no one knows how to keep people from developing leukemia. For most forms of leukemia, there is nothing about the way a person lives that puts them at risk for developing the disease. But as we have already discussed, where you live and what you are exposed to may put you at a higher risk for developing the illness. Unfortunately, most people do not realize that they live in a high-risk area until people around them begin to show signs of illness, and by then it is too late. However, these environmental risk factors are believed to cause only a small number of the cases of leukemia.

Acute leukemia is the type of leukemia most often linked to environmental causes such as radiation and chemical exposure. Oddly enough, as you will learn later, radiation and chemotherapy are also ways of treating leukemia and other cancers. Of course, one of the bad things about these treatments is that they can also cause cancer. It can be a vicious cycle, so your doctors must be very careful when they decide which treatments to give you.

An important thing to keep in mind is that if you have leukemia, it is no one's fault. No one gave it to you. You did not catch it from someone else who has it, nor did you inherit it from your mom or dad. There is nothing you could have done differently in your past that would have kept you from getting leukemia. It is not your fault that you have leukemia. It is no one's fault, which is why concentrating on your treatment is the best thing you can do for yourself and your body.

The Hospital

Following a diagnosis of leukemia, your doctor may want you to check into the hospital for a while because he or she may want to keep an eye on you and monitor your health. Most likely you will go into the hospital to receive treatments such as radiation therapy or chemotherapy, which will be discussed in detail in chapter 5 and chapter 6. Some children spend more time in the hospital than other children do. Like the illness itself, how much time a person spends in the hospital will depend upon each individual. It may help if you know what to expect at the hospital before you actually go there.

"I was really scared the first time I had to go into the hospital," says Tara, fourteen. "I had never been away from my family for more than one night. But the hospital let my mom stay with me and my friends were allowed to visit me, too. I liked my nurses and there was even a teen room that I could go to where I got to do art projects and stuff."

Can My Mom or Dad Stay?

It should be fine for your mom or dad to stay with you at the hospital, even overnight. You may be able to have your parent stay right there in your room with you, or accommodations may be made for your parent to stay in a room close by. If you are feeling well and up to having company, your relatives and friends can come to visit you. Each hospital has its own rules and guidelines regarding visitors. It will be best to check with your nurse before anyone comes up to visit. Also, you will want to discourage visitors from coming to visit you if they are sick or not feeling well, as you are going to be more susceptible to their infections. Your immune system is already having a hard time doing its job for you.

At this point, catching something like a cold or the flu can really make you sick.

When You First Get There

When you first get to the hospital, you will be shown to your room. It may be a private room, or you may have to share it with one or more other patients. You will probably have an IV placed in one of your arms. This will provide a way for medicines to be delivered right into your body. You will probably get started on your treatments right away. You may go for X rays or other tests. There may be a lot to do when you are in the hospital. Try to relax and just go with it. Everything is being done to help you get well.

Doctors and Nurses

Doctors are the people who will examine you, make the diagnosis, prescribe treatment, and ask you how you are doing. They have your best interests in mind, and they want to do everything in their power to help you get well as soon as possible.

Nurses are the men and women who are available around the clock to help you out. They will bring your medicines, answer your questions, and make sure everything you need is taken care of. They work very hard and they may be taking care of several people at one time, so be patient. However, if you have an emergency or you honestly feel that you are not being well taken care of, you have the right to ask for further assistance.

Also as a patient, you have the right to ask questions about anything you are unsure of or need to understand better. Do not be afraid to ask questions about your health status or your care. If you are not sure about something, ask. If you do not understand something, ask. There are no stupid questions. This is your body we are talking about. You have the right to know what is going on.

Will I Get Any Sleep?

When you are sick, you need more sleep than you do when you are healthy. On your first night in the hospital, you will probably notice noises that you are unfamiliar with, and they may keep you awake. Nurses may come in throughout the night to check your vital signs, such as your temperature and your blood pressure. Eventually you will adjust to your new surroundings and you will get used to the strange noises and the interruptions.

How Will I Feel and What Will I Do?

Some of the medicines and treatments you receive in the hospital may make you feel worse than you did when you first got there. It is true that you often have to feel worse before you feel better. When you are feeling good, however, you can do your homework, read, watch videos, or play games. There may even be a special room or area for kids to hang out and talk. Every hospital is different and each offers different services to the patients. Ask your nurse if there are any special programs offered in your hospital.

Chemotherapy

This chapter will talk about chemotherapy, also referred to as chemo, one of the main methods of fighting cancer. While you are reading about the ways to treat leukemia, remember that your doctor will not recommend any treatment unless the benefits, like controlling your leukemia and relieving its symptoms, outweigh the known risks of the treatment. He or she will not suggest any treatment that is likely to make you far sicker than you are already. Your doctor has in mind both your short–term health and your long–term health, and will do his or her best to help you get as healthy as possible. Optimally, you will return to your normal, preleukemia state of health with few or no remaining side effects.

What Is Chemotherapy?

When you hear the word "chemo," what images come to mind? If you have ever heard about someone who has had to have chemo, you may think about the person losing his or her hair and vomiting a lot. So chemo is a pretty scary word to hear. However, it could also be the treatment that makes your leukemia go away. Let's get to know something about chemo so that it is not such a frightening subject.

Leukemia was the first type of cancer that was controlled by chemotherapy. The word "chemotherapy" really just means drugs used to treat a disease. It is one of the two main ways that cancer is treated. (The other way is called radiation, and we will talk about that in chapter 6.) Doctors administer combinations of drugs based on the type of cancer a person has and the stage of the cancer. Although chemo may not cure your cancer, it may be your best defense against it. With some forms of cancer, chemo may keep it under control for a long time, even if it does not make it go away. Chemo may be used by itself or with radiation treatments or surgery, depending on what your doctor thinks is the best treatment for you.

Children and teens that have acute lymphocytic leukemia will almost always start their first course of chemo as soon as a definite diagnosis of leukemia is made.

Will I Lose My Hair?

So what exactly happens when your doctor decides that you should have chemo? There are a great number of different drugs that are used in this treatment. Various drugs work in different ways, but they all work toward the same goal, which is keeping the cancer cells from reproducing. The side effects you will experience are also going to be pretty much the same. If you are going to have chemo, you can expect to experience the following side effects: vomiting, hair loss, loss of appetite, tiredness, nausea, diarrhea, and suppressed bone marrow function.

You are probably most familiar with the first two symptoms on the list. Everyone throws up at one time or another, usually when they have the flu. The reason that you throw up when you have chemo is because it reacts with your intestines, as well as with the center in your brain that controls such reactions. Luckily, your doctor can prescribe other medicines that you can take that will keep you from vomiting.

"They gave me some medicine that I could take to help me in case I felt like I was going to throw up," says Kat, now twenty and in remission for two years, *"but I never really felt like I had to throw up. Some people just don't throw up.*

"Losing my hair was pretty weird though. Actually, I didn't want to watch it all fall out, so about a week after I found out that my hair would be falling out, I shaved my head. It started growing back a few months later, after I'd finished chemo and was nearing the end of my radiation treatments.

"My head got cold at night, but other than that, losing my hair really was not all that bad. The hardest part was when people would stare at me. Sometimes people would ask me why I was bald and then they would get scared when I told them the reason. That was hard, too.

"The weirdest thing that ever happened because I had no hair was the time a little girl told me I looked like an alien. That was really bizarre. Other than that, being bald did not really bother me. My cousins thought I looked really cute. When my hair did finally start to grow back, it came in different from the way it had been before I got sick. It was curly."

Throwing up may not seem like a big deal to you. On the other hand, you might find the idea of losing your hair to be quite upsetting. One thing to remember is that your hair will grow back. Most people discover that losing their hair is a small price to pay for getting better.

Other Side Effects

Another set of chemo-related side effects is caused by the fact that chemo may kill off some of your body's healthy cells along with the leukemia cells. These side effects have to do with your blood because some of your developing blood cells get killed along with the leukemia cells. This may lead to anemia, which you already know is a severe deficiency of red blood cells. Severe deficiencies in phagocytes—cells that surround foreign bodies and other unwanted materials—result in blood cell deficiencies like neutropenia, monocytopenia, and thrombocytopenia. These conditions are serious because they can result in other health problems, such as excessive bleeding, anemia, and bacterial or fungal infections, which require antibiotics. Some symptoms that may indicate that you have an infection are fever, chills, cough, soreness or tenderness in a particular area of your body, sore throat, pain when you urinate, and diarrhea.

If you develop any of these blood cell deficiencies, you may need to have a blood transfusion. You may need only red blood cells or platelets, depending on what component of your blood is low. If, for example, your neutrophils and monocytes are low, you will only be able to take antibiotics, as there is no method yet available to transfuse these cells. As your body gets rid of the leukemia cells and new, healthy blood cells are allowed to grow normally, you will no longer need to have blood transfusions or take antibiotics.

The War Against Infection

Until your body is free of leukemia and the added risk of infection, there are things that you can do to help your body avoid infection. Always wash your hands when you are ready to eat, after you have been out in public or with other people, and especially after going to the bathroom. Make sure that the people taking care of you, like your family, doctors, nurses, and therapists, also wash their hands before they touch you. Ask your friends to wash their hands before they handle your things or come in contact with you. Hand washing may seem like a small task, but it is a small step that can prevent a huge problem.

As we discussed, your gums are a prime place for infection. Be sure to pay close attention to your oral hygiene when you have leukemia. Your dentist can assist you in working out a dental care plan that will keep your gums and teeth as healthy as possible.

How Does Chemo Work?

The drugs used in chemotherapy affect cells in the body that divide rapidly, which is what cancer cells do. However, other cells in the body besides the cancer cells divide rapidly as well. These are the cells of your hair follicles, mouth, skin, stomach, intestines, and bone marrow. This is why you experience side effects.

If the side effects you experience are much more than your body can handle, your doctor can try different combinations of drugs or stop the drug therapy for a short period of time, giving your body a chance to rest. Remember that all of the symptoms associated with chemo are temporary. As soon as your chemo is done, the side effects will go away. Depending on how you feel while you are getting chemo, you may be able to go on with your normal activities. Some people never suffer from any of the side effects of chemo.

There are a few different ways that chemotherapy drugs can be given. The most common ways are by mouth and by injection. When chemo drugs are injected, they go straight into a muscle or vein in your body. They are usually given for a few days in a row and then you get a few days off for rest. Then you will go back and get another cycle of chemo. This method has been found to be the best way to let your body's normal cells have a fair chance to recover and function.

As mentioned earlier, chemo cannot distinguish between healthy cells and cancer cells, so any cells that are rapid dividers are targets of the chemo drugs. So, while the hope is that the chemo will kill off the cancer cells, it kills off some healthy cells as well. The resting time between doses of chemo gives your healthy cells a chance for survival.

Where Do I Receive Chemotherapy Treatments?

Chemo is usually given at the hospital or at a hospital clinic. Depending on certain factors—where you live in relation to the hospital and how sick you are—you may go to the hospital every day during the course of your chemo, get your treatment, and go home. Or you may check into the hospital for a few days to receive your chemo. You may also have a prescription for some oral medication, which you will be able to take at home.

"When I was getting chemo I had to be at the hospital at 9:00 in the morning," says Kat. "First I had to have my blood tested to see if my count was high enough to get chemo. The results would come back around noon. If my counts were okay, I would go in and start the chemo. It took about two hours. There were two pushes. Pushes are just medications that are pushed into the IV line by a nurse. I had one IV medicine that took about twenty minutes, and another IV drip that took an hour. Basically getting chemo was an all-day affair."

If you are going to have chemo, your doctor will probably want you to have an indwelling catheter, a small tube that provides easy access to your veins, placed in a vein in your upper chest. The alternative is getting pricked with a needle every time blood has to be drawn or medicines have to be given, leaving your veins bruised and sore. Without an indwelling catheter, it becomes hard to find a vein that is still strong enough to be poked, so having it eliminates the need to poke many different areas of your body. The indwelling catheter is fairly discreet and most people will not even know that you have it. Whenever you need to receive medicine or blood, or have your blood drawn for testing, your indwelling catheter will provide easy access.

Chemo and Other Meds

When you are getting chemo, your body may be extra-sensitive to certain things such as infection and other drugs. It is important that you talk to your doctor about things that you should and should not do when you are having chemo. For example, your body's resistance to infections may become lower when you are having chemo, so it will be especially important for you to try to stay away from people who are sick with the flu or a cold. If you catch either of these, you will be sicker than the person you caught it from.

You can eat what you want unless your doctor has put you on a special diet, and you can do all of your regular activities if you feel well enough to do them. However, you should not take any other medicines, even vitamins, aspirin, or birth control pills, unless you have had a discussion with your doctor and he or she agrees to let you take these medications. If you have other questions about chemo and what you can and cannot do when you are on it, you should talk to your doctor. He or she will help you decide what is safe for you and what activities you should avoid.

New Drugs Coming Soon

New drugs to fight different kinds of cancers are being researched and developed all the time. Sometimes a new drug is offered in another country that has not been approved in the United States. The United States has very strict rules and regulations about drug testing and use. Drugs take several years to gain approval and make their way to the public.

When scientists discover or develop a new cancer-fighting drug, many steps must be taken to determine whether or not the drug works and is safe for people to take. Scientists begin by trying the drugs out on animals that have been specially bred and raised to do this kind of important work. First, the animals are given cancer, and then they are injected with the new drug. The animals' reactions to the new drug are very important, as this will give scientists information about how humans will react to the medication.

Scientists use what they learn to determine the dose needed to fight cancer cells without damaging too many healthy tissues and cells. Once these things have been checked out, the new drug has to be approved by the Federal Drug Administration (FDA).

After the drug is tested on animals and determined to be safe by the FDA, it still has to be tested on people. When you are going through chemotherapy, your doctor may suggest a new experimental drug or explain that there is a drug trial going on that you may qualify to take part in. The new drug may hold the key to your recovery and you will also be helping other people who get sick with leukemia in the future. Your participation in the drug trial will help doctors prescribe the drug to future patients, and you will know that you have helped other people get well.

Most drug studies involve many patients, some of whom receive the actual drug and the rest of whom receive a placebo, which looks just like the real drug but contains no medicine. If you take part in this type of test, you will not know whether you have received treatment until the test is completed. For this reason, participating in a drug study is not the best choice for everyone. Your doctor will determine whether you are a good candidate for participation.

The process of bringing a new drug to the market can take several years. These years are necessary for ensuring that the new drug does not cause people to suffer needlessly because the drug is not being used properly or will cause bad effects later on. These precautions are for your own safety. Your doctor will give you a drug only if he or she believes it will be effective in fighting your leukemia with absolute safety.

Other Options

Researchers continue to work on developing new medicines that will fight leukemia. They are testing new synthetic drugs, meaning drugs created in a laboratory, and new natural drugs, which are drugs found in nature or created using natural sources.

Researchers are also trying out new and different combinations of drugs that have already proven effective in fighting leukemia and other forms of cancer. Immunotherapy is a possible treatment of the future.

With immunotherapy, the body's natural defenses are made stronger so that they can prevent or kill the leukemia cells. One example of immunotherapy is called radioimmunotherapy, in which antibodies—proteins produced by the body that neutralize or react with antigens—that emit radiation are injected into the leukemia patient. Once they are in the body they get to work destroying leukemia cells. Another approach to immunotherapy involves the use of normal lymphocytes that have been immunized. The immune lymphocytes do not recognize leukemia cells, meaning they think the leukemia cells are foreign bodies that must be attacked and killed off.

Radiation Therapy

"Radiation was really not that bad," says Kat. "I just had to lie down on a big table and I could not move until they told me it was okay. They had to give me a small tattoo mark on my chest. It is only a dot, but it marked the center of where they were supposed to put the radiation."

Radiation therapy is another method of treatment, sometimes called radiotherapy, X-ray therapy, or irradiation. This type of therapy treats cancer by using penetrating beams of high-energy waves or streams of particles that are called radiation.

How Does Radiation Treatment Work?

A long time ago, doctors discovered that they could use radiation to look inside the human body and find disease. This is known today as an X ray, and uses relatively low, safe doses of radiation. Higher doses of radiation, doctors later discovered, could be used to treat cancer.

A machine containing radiation aims specific amounts of radiation beams at the cancer in your body, and the high doses of radiation work by killing off the cancer cells or preventing them from growing and dividing further. As you already know, cancer cells grow and divide more rapidly than most of the normal cells around them. Radiation therapy catches those faster cells and literally zaps them. Unfortunately, as with chemotherapy, some of your normal cells will also be affected by the radiation. Luckily, however, most of the normal cells will be able to recover from the bad effects of the radiation, unlike the cancer cells, which do not recover and die off.

The goal of radiation therapy is to kill the cancer cells without causing any major damage to your normal cells. Your doctor will do as much as possible to protect your normal, healthy cells. By carefully limiting the doses of radiation, spreading out treatments over time, and shielding as much of your normal tissue as possible, your normal cells have the best chance of recovering and staying healthy. More than half of all people who have cancer of some kind are treated with some form of radiation therapy. For some people who have cancer, radiation is the only kind of treatment they will need.

Combination Treatments

Radiation treatment affects cancer cells only in a specific area of the body. Sometimes doctors add radiation therapy to treatments like chemotherapy that reach all parts of the body. The combination of the two treatments might make your chances of recovery even better.

Other times, radiation therapy may be used along with surgery to treat cancer. For example, doctors may give a person radiation therapy before surgery to shrink a tumor because it may be easier to remove a small tumor than a large one. The surgery will then be less extensive. Radiation therapy may also be used following surgery to stop the growth of cancer cells that may have been left behind.

Your doctors will be very careful to get the combination of radiation and chemotherapy just right for your illness and for your body. Radiation treatment given before or during chemotherapy will reduce the number of cancer cells so that there are fewer for chemotherapy to destroy. Radiation treatment following chemotherapy will be given to make a "final sweep" of your body to clear out any remaining cancer cells that did not get destroyed when you were having chemo treatments.

Some Important Facts About Radiation Therapy

The side effects that you experience from the radiation treatments are almost all temporary. There are a few risks involved, but they are all for the greater good of killing off the cancer in your body.

- Radiation treatments do not hurt.

- Radiation therapy will not make you radioactive.

- Radiation treatments are usually scheduled every day except weekends.

- Radiation sessions take about thirty minutes each, although the actual radiation treatment takes only a few minutes.

⇨ You should try hard to get enough sleep and also try to eat well-balanced meals while you are undergoing radiation therapy.

⇨ The area of skin at which the radiation is aimed may become red, sensitive, and easily irritated.

How Is Radiation Therapy Given?

Radiation treatments are normally given on an outpatient basis, meaning that you do not have to actually check in and stay at the hospital to get your radiation therapy. Instead, you can go to the hospital or clinic every day and then go back home or off to school when you are done with the session.

A radiation therapy machine directs high-energy rays of radiation at the cancer and a small bit of the surrounding area. There are several different types of machines used for radiation. Each machine works in a slightly different way and is used depending on the type of cancer and its location in a person's body. Your doctor will make the decision as to which machine is the right one for you.

Your cancer doctor, or oncologist, will work with a radiation oncologist to organize your radiation treatments. A radiation oncologist is a doctor who specializes in using radiation to treat cancer. The radiation oncologist will work very closely with all of the other doctors and health care professionals who are on your health care team. He or she will prescribe the type of radiation you will receive and decide the amount of radiation that will work well for you.

What Do I Have to Do?

When you arrive for your radiation therapy, you will be given a hospital gown to change into. Your radiation therapist will then look for the marks that have been tattooed onto your skin. These marks tell him or her exactly where the radiation has to go into your body. Next, you will either lie down on a treatment table or sit in a treatment chair and the radiation therapist will place a lead shield over your body to protect your healthy organs and other healthy tissues during radiation. There might also be plastic or plaster forms that help you stay still. The radiation must go to the exact same spot every time. You will be in the radiation treatment room for about fifteen to thirty minutes, but your actual dose of radiation will take only about one to five minutes.

Receiving radiation treatments does not hurt. In fact, it will not seem much different from having an X ray taken. You will probably not even know when you are getting the radiation because you will not be able to hear, see, or smell it.

While you are receiving the treatments, the radiation therapist will leave and work the radiation machine from a nearby room. The therapist will keep a close eye on you from a window in the machine control room or from a television screen. If you start to feel lonely or afraid while you are getting your radiation treatment, remember that the radiation therapist is right in the next room. In fact, there will probably be an intercom through which you can talk if you have any problems. So if you start to feel sick or especially uncomfortable while you are getting your treatment, you can tell the therapist right away, and the radiation machine can be stopped.

The actual machines that dispense the radiation are very large. They make loud, strange noises as they move around your body aiming the radiation into the right spots in your body from different angles. At first this may seem frightening, but eventually you will get so used to it that you will not even notice the noise.

"I used to close my eyes," says Kat, "and pretend that I was on a beach in Hawaii. I would pretend that the noise I was hearing was really the waves lapping up on the shore. I got so good at this that sometimes the radiation therapist had to come in and tell me that the time was up and that I could leave."

How Long Does Radiation Take?

Radiation therapy is usually given for six or seven weeks, Monday through Friday, with weekends off. The reason the treatment takes so long is that your doctor is trying to protect the rest of your body from the harmful effects of the radiation. By giving you small amounts, your healthy cells have a chance to recover in between radiation doses.

One very important thing to remember is that skipping a session is bad news. If you skip or miss too many radiation therapy sessions, you are doing yourself a great disservice. You will not get well unless you follow your doctor's instructions, so if you do not make it to all of your scheduled radiation therapy sessions, you are only cheating yourself. Of course, if there is an emergency situation that arises, this can be dealt with. But you have to let your doctor know what is going on so that you can make arrangements to make up the sessions that you have missed.

A Few Radiation Tips to Remember

You may want to take a few precautions to protect your body while you are going through your treatment sessions. You can really help yourself by eating a well-balanced diet and maintaining proper nutrition. Now is not the time to be on a diet. If you need help planning good meals, you can talk to your nurse or a nutritionist. Along similar lines, do not take vitamins or herbal preparations without first talking to your doctor.

Taking special care of your skin, especially the treated area, is also a good idea. Check with your doctor or nurse about the things you may be putting on your skin. You should ask if there are special products that you should be using. The following things can irritate your skin on the treatment area: soap and bath gel, body lotion, deodorant, makeup, shaving lotion or cream, bandages, ice packs, heating pads, and hot water. Your skin may also be extra sensitive to the clothing material that you normally wear, as well as to detergents and fabric softeners.

A Word About the Sun

During radiation treatments, you need to be especially careful about protecting your sensitive skin. The area on which you receive the radiation must be kept from sun exposure. When you have to go outside in the sun, wear light-colored clothes to protect your skin. Talk to your doctor about whether or not you should also be using sunscreen or a sunblock lotion, and how soon following a radiation treatment it is safe to apply it. If your doctor wants you to use a product to protect your skin from the sun, choose one that has a sun protection factor (SPF) of at least 15. Be sure to apply it carefully, covering all exposed skin, and reapply it often if you are staying outside for a substantial length of time. These are just some basic sun protection guidelines. If you have any more questions about the sun, you can ask your doctor or nurse.

Bone Marrow Transplants

Another treatment available for fighting leukemia is the bone marrow transplant. Bone marrow transplants are still considered to be a relatively new form of treatment for leukemia, even though the first successful transplant was done in 1968.

Your doctor will let you know if you could benefit from a bone marrow transplant because not all leukemia will respond to a transplant. Also, not everyone who needs a bone marrow transplant actually gets one. This is unfortunate, because for some people a bone marrow transplant offers the very best chance for recovery. However, there are certain criteria that must be met before a person can receive one. With all of these sobering facts in mind, let us look into the specifics of a bone marrow transplant.

Blood and Bone Marrow

Blood is made of two main components, cells and plasma. The cells, which you already know about, are red blood cells, platelets, white blood cells, eosinophils, basophils, and lymphocytes. All of these cells are suspended in plasma, which is mostly water. Many of the chemicals found naturally in your body are dissolved in this plasma. These chemicals are things like proteins, hormones, vitamins and minerals, and antibodies.

All of the blood cells in your bone marrow start out as stem cells—the cells that grow up and turn into the different types of cells that make up your blood. This process is called differentiation. When you were healthy, your stem cells were great enough in number to keep the continuous process of blood production in your body moving along at a normal pace. The stem cells branched off first into two different types of cells called multipotential hematopoietic cells and multipotential lymphocytic cells. The multipotential hematopoietic cells differentiate and mature to become the six types of blood cells. The multipotential lymphocytic cells differentiate and mature to become lymphocytes: T cells, B cells, and natural killer cells. All of these cells, which get their start in your bone marrow, move out into your bloodstream and into the rest of your tissues, doing their different jobs to keep you healthy and alive.

As you already know, if you have leukemia, some of these complex functions are not working right. One way to fix this, depending on which type of leukemia you have, is to give you some brand-new, healthy bone marrow from which new and healthy stem cells can start growing. By giving you healthy new stem cells, your body has a better chance of growing healthy mature cells. You may hear stem cell transplants being referred to as SCTs and bone marrow transplants being called BMTs, although both mean almost the same thing.

How Would a BMT Help Me?

All blood cells are produced by stem cells. However, if your stem cells are sick and not behaving properly, you can get rid of them and replace them with new, healthy stem cells.

You may be wondering where these "new" stem cells come from. Extra stem cells are constantly circulating throughout your bloodstream. There are not many of them there, but your doctor can give you special drugs that will make the number of stem cells in your blood increase by drawing them out of your bone marrow. Then your doctor will take some of the blood from your body and circulate it through a machine called a hemapheresis machine. This machine skims off the blood cells that have stems cells in them. This process is called recovering stem cells for transplant. If your own bone marrow is used to treat your leukemia it is called an autologous transplant.

The other place that new stem cells or bone marrow come from is another person. This is called an allogenic bone marrow transplant. The person most likely to give you his or her bone marrow is one of your brothers or sisters. Your siblings' genetic makeup is closest to matching yours, making them the people who are most likely to have the same or most similar tissue makeup. What this means is that there are certain components of your blood that have to match up to your donor's blood. Your brother or sister is more likely than anyone else to have the same components as you do because you share the same parents. If you do not have a brother or a sister, your parents are your next best chance for a match. After your parents, other relatives will be considered. Of course, unless you have an identical twin, there remains the possibility that no one in your family is a perfect match for you. You may have to go with a family member who is a partial match, or you may need to look outside your family for a bone marrow match.

Searching for a Non-Related Donor

The National Marrow Donor Program is a national clear-inghouse of people who have voluntarily donated a sample of their blood in hopes of becoming a match for someone who needs a bone marrow transplant. Thousands of people need bone marrow transplants every year and not all of those people can find a match within their own families. Finding an unrelated match without an organization set up for this very purpose was a nearly impossible task, so in 1987, the National Marrow Donor Program set up a computerized data bank of thousands of available tissue-typed donors from all over the country. Now, anyone in need of a bone marrow donor can contact the National Marrow Donor Program and follow the procedures to search for a potential match.

Your blood will be tested to find out your Human Leukocyte Antigen (HLA) type, also known as your tissue type. HLA type is similar to blood type in that just as you would have to match the blood type of someone whose blood was being transfused into your body, so you also need to match the HLA type of someone whose bone marrow you are about to receive. HLA type is a way of classifying people according to markers on the surface of their white blood cells. The donor's HLA type and yours must match if a transplant is going to be made. If the HLA types do not match, there is no chance of the bone marrow transplant working for you.

If a potential match is located through the National Marrow Donor Program computer system, he or she will be contacted and more tests will be done to determine whether or not this person is actually a suitable match for you. This volunteer will also have a chance to decide whether or not he or she truly wants to become a bone marrow donor. He or she still has the right and the option to change his or her mind. There comes a point, however, after your match has agreed to become your donor, that he or she is morally obligated to donate his or her marrow because for you there is no turning back.

If your doctor has determined that your type of leukemia would benefit from a bone marrow transplant, you may want to take matters into your own hands, especially if you have already checked with the National Marrow Donor Program and found out that there is no current match for you. The National Marrow Donor Program can help your family, friends, and neighbors organize their own bone marrow donor drive.

"I don't have any brothers or sisters and no one else in my family was a good enough match for me," says Alana, fourteen. *"So we went to the National Marrow Donor Program for help, but we couldn't find a match there either. I was getting sicker and sicker and I was getting scared that I would die.*

The National Marrow Donor Program suggested

we have a bone marrow donor drive of our own. We printed up posters with my picture on it. We had a bunch of friends help us put them up all over the neighborhood, so people would know that we were having the drive. One company donated a bunch of stuff so we had T-shirts, buttons, and balloons, too.

"The drive was on two different weekends, and they were held at my school. Practically everyone we knew showed up. In fact, over the two weekends we had about 500 people come. It made me feel really good that all of these people cared so much about me that they came out to help. And I also knew that even if I didn't find a donor for myself, someone else might. The most exciting part of our drive was that I did find a donor and I am doing really great now."

What Are the Chances of Finding a Match for a BMT?

Your best chance of finding a match is if someone in your family has the same HLA type as you do. But only about 30 percent of people who need bone marrow transplants actually find a match within their family. The chances of two unrelated people having matching HLA types are about 1 in 20,000. The more people who are registered in the National Marrow Donor Program, the more chances you have of finding a match.

No Turning Back

Once a suitable HLA match has been located for you and your match has agreed to become your donor, you will have to go through some very serious procedures. After some preliminary steps, such as talking to your doctor about why you need the transplant, and learning how your body may react, you will have to go into protective isolation in the hospital. Soon after, the bone marrow that is causing your body so much trouble will be removed from your body. A combination of radiation and chemotherapy treatments will be used to destroy all of the bone marrow in your body. When your body is completely free of all traces of bone marrow, you have reached the point where there is no turning back.

You cannot live without bone marrow, so at this point you have no choice but to get the transplant. The new, healthy bone marrow from your donor will be transplanted into your body as soon as your diseased bone marrow has been completely destroyed.

When you receive your bone marrow transplant, the marrow moves into your bloodstream and your body gets to work. The new marrow naturally grafts itself into your bones, filling the space where your diseased bone marrow used to be. When your doctor tests your blood and finds that your white blood cell count has gone up, you have evidence that the graft has happened. Your white count will continue to increase and your body will begin to produce new platelets, too. After four to six weeks have passed, you will be able to come out of protective isolation and go back to a regular hospital room where you will be able to receive visitors. Ideally, your health will continue to improve and you will eventually be able to go back to school and do all of the things that you were doing before you got sick.

Could Something Go Wrong?

There are no guarantees. Your transplant should be a success, but your doctor will explain to you the possible problems that may arise. You have to remain optimistic and hope for the best. After all, you would not have gone through the transplant procedure if you did not believe that it would do you a great deal of good. Still, there are no guarantees that the bone marrow transplant will be a complete success.

The most common problem that occurs is rejection. Rejection, in this case, is what happens when your body does not accept the new bone marrow the way it should. No graft has occurred. Your new bone marrow is not going to get the job done. Another problem is known as graft-versus-host disease, and this occurs when your new marrow gets into a fight with your body. You could also get an infection because your entire immune system was essentially destroyed when your bone marrow was drained, leaving you more susceptible. The last complication is that you could have a relapse. Even if the new bone marrow does graft to your body, the leukemia might come back again. Although any of these complications can occur, in most cases they can be treated, giving you a better chance of recovery.

How Do I Volunteer to Be a Donor?

If you know people who meet the following requirements, encourage them to join the National Marrow Donor Program: Marrow donors must be between the ages of eighteen and fifty-five and they must be in good enough health to pass a physical exam.

Becoming a member of the National Marrow Donor Program does not cost the donor anything at all. All someone has to do is give two tablespoons of blood, sign a consent form, and then go back to his or her regular routine and hope to be called. The blood sample the person gives will be HLA-typed at a medical lab, and the results will be cataloged in the National Marrow Donor Program's computer so that searches can be made from all over the country.

Few people are actually called and told that they are a preliminary match for someone who needs a bone marrow transplant. However, if a person does get a call, he or she will have to get a bit more blood drawn for further testing. If he or she is an exact match, counselors and doctors will talk to the donor, explaining the need for his or her bone marrow and the procedure used to get it. Basically, the potential donor will receive all of the information he or she needs to make an informed decision.

Once the donor has made a commitment and the recipient has undergone chemo and radiation in preparation for receiving the new bone marrow, the life of the leukemia patient is in the hands of the donor. You understand the depth of this commitment because you have already read about it in the previous section.

The Donor's Role

You are in luck. A volunteer whose HLA type matches yours has been found and has agreed to become your bone marrow donor. Now what happens?

Your donor will be treated with special care because he or she is about to provide you with a healthy life once again. He or she will not be asked to make any life changes, such as diet or work habits. However, for your benefit, your donor may be asked to avoid taking any unnecessary risks that could cause him or her to get hurt or sick.

The next step is for your donor to go into the hospital, but not necessarily the same hospital that you are in. In fact, depending on the wishes of your donor and where he or she lives in relation to where you live, you may or may not ever meet. Your donor will be told that you need his or her bone marrow in order to get well, but that is about all the donor will learn about you. However, your donor will be invited to contact a program coordinator to get updates on you and how well you are doing. Your donor will not be able to contact you personally, but he or she can let the coordinator know that he or she would like to be contacted, if you so desire. If you want to contact your donor, you can talk to your coordinator who can help you to arrange contact between you and your donor, if your donor is willing. Overall, contact must be mutual.

Extracting the Donor's Bone Marrow

Your donor will receive anesthesia either at the site of incision, called a local anesthetic, or a general anesthetic, which will put him or her to sleep for the duration of the procedure. Four or eight very small incisions will be made in the back pelvic area, near the pelvic bones at both sides of the lower back. About 5 to 10 percent of your donor's bone marrow is removed from these incisions. Using a large syringe to draw out the marrow, the whole procedure usually takes about forty-five to sixty minutes.

67

All of this is done in the safe and sterile atmosphere of a hospital. Your donor will stay in the hospital for either a few hours or overnight, but then he or she will be able to go home. Of course, the donor's lower back may be sore for a few days after the bone marrow donation. But surely he or she will feel that this bit of discomfort is a small price to pay for helping you out in such a major way.

After the marrow has been collected from your donor, it is sent without delay to the hospital where you are waiting. You will have an IV already in place when the bone marrow arrives, and you will go through a procedure that is pretty similar to a blood transfusion. It will not hurt you at all to receive your bone marrow transplant.

Taking Care
of Yourself

If you have been diagnosed with leukemia, you will want to know how it is going to affect your everyday life. At this point we have discussed things like being in the hospital, treatment options, the side effects of treatments, and bone marrow transplants. It all seems pretty complicated and by now you are probably thinking that you are about to spend the rest of your life being sick. Although this may be the picture in your mind, it is not reality. In fact, many children and teens who get leukemia continue to live their lives as they did before they were diagnosed. Of course, there will be trips to the hospital, blood tests, and treatments, but in between all of these things you may be able to do many of the things you would normally be doing, like going to school, dating, hanging out with friends, and preparing for your future.

You should expect to feel better on some days than you feel on other days. On the good days you may feel like doing everything. On the bad days you may not even want to get out of bed. A combination of good days and bad days is pretty typical for any person suffering from a serious illness. The important thing to remember is that you and your doctors are working hard to get you back to your original, good state of health. So even if you are feeling pretty lousy right now, the good, healthy days are ahead for you once again. Stick it out.

Healthy Habits Make a Healthy Person

Although your doctors are working hard to choose the right medicines for you and you are getting the best care possible, you can also do some things for yourself as well. Healthy people know that they will be even healthier if they exercise, eat right, get enough sleep, and avoid too much stress. The same is true for people who have leukemia.

Exercise

Exercising to keep your body in shape is always a good idea. You may like to go to a gym and do aerobics or lift weights. You may run on your school's track team or play basketball in your neighborhood park every day after school. You know how good you feel when your exercise session is complete. Unless your doctor tells you not to, you should be able to continue to exercise as you normally would, but it is very important for you to check with your doctor first.

For one reason or another you may be advised against exercising, or you may be advised to change your exercise routine to a milder, less strenuous routine. If your doctor suggests that you should tone down your workouts, follow the advice. It is for your own good. Exercise is good only if it is going to help you. If your doctor feels that exercising may do your body more harm than good, you need to listen to what you are being told and adapt your exercise routine to meet the needs of your body while you have leukemia.

You may also find that you are just too tired to exercise like you once did. This is not an unusual side effect of leukemia and the treatments you are going through. If you do not feel up to exercising the way you normally would, ask yourself if there is something else you can do instead. For example, if you used to run a few miles a day, perhaps you could take a casual walk instead. Or if you are used to playing basketball for two hours after school, maybe you could play for just half an hour and then take a break. It is extremely important to listen to your body and the signals it is sending out. Now is not the time to push yourself to make the team or go the extra mile. There will be plenty of time for that once you are well again. And once again, it must be stressed: Listen to your body. If your body is telling you that you need to rest, you should rest.

Eating Right

You should be able to eat all of your favorite foods when you have leukemia. There is not a special leukemia diet. However, like exercise, eating right and on a regular basis will help your body feel better overall. Eating well-balanced meals will help you keep up your energy and give your body the extra fuel it needs for its fight to get well.

Getting enough food is also important right now. Unless your doctor specifically recommends that you diet, now is not the time to be worrying about your weight. Your doctor or a nutritionist can help you choose foods that are high in iron and other foods that will help you feel good and keep your body healthy. Of course, you can still have an occasional candy bar and potato chips, but a steady diet of junk food will not help you fight leukemia.

Depending on the treatments you are taking and the degree of your illness, you may not feel like eating. This can be rather frustrating, especially since you know you need to eat. If you do not feel like eating, you may start to lose weight. When you lose weight, your body has less of a reserve to help it fight the disease. Again, your doctor or nutritionist can help you find foods that appeal to you and also suggest some high calorie, high nutrition dietary supplements.

You should also be taking vitamins right now, but again, check with your doctor first. He or she may want you to take specific vitamins, depending on the medications you are taking.

Get Enough Sleep

You have probably already noticed that having leukemia makes you tired. In fact, being extra tired might have been one of the first symptoms that led you to your diagnosis. If you are tired, this is your body's way of saying you need extra sleep. While you sleep, your body works hard to repair the everyday damage that occurs while you are awake. As your body fights the leukemia, you may run out of energy faster than usual. You may feel especially run-down and tired. Once again, listen to what your body is telling you. If you feel tired, sleep.

Some of your medications may also make you feel especially sleepy. Your doctor may be able to give you a different medication or a medication that counteracts this effect. But again, if you are tired, go ahead and go to bed. This is not the time to be pushing yourself.

Pulling all-nighters to finish a paper or study for a test or partying with your friends late into the night is not recommended. Your friends have to understand that while you are sick you have limits. Pushing your body beyond those limits by not getting the sleep your body needs to fight your disease can actually harm you further. Your immune system will begin to waiver even more if you are not getting a proper amount of sleep. All teens love to sleep. Now you have a great excuse to sleep all you want to. Indulge yourself. It will actually help you this time.

Avoid Too Much Stress

This is probably the most difficult of all the healthy recommendations suggested in this section. Having an illness such as leukemia can make for a highly stressful situation. You already know that. You and your family have probably already felt stressed out quite a bit. It is going to be nearly impossible to avoid all stress at this time, but you can avoid certain stresses. For example, if you know you have a paper due or a test coming up, start preparing early rather than leaving things to the last minute. If you have certain friends who routinely stress you out, perhaps you will want to spend a bit less time with them.

Now is not the time to take on any added responsibilities. Although you should continue with your usual activities, if you are already working part-time after school and serving on the yearbook committee at school, now may not be the time to add drama club and student council to your schedule. In fact, you may actually find yourself having to choose between your after-school job and the yearbook committee. You just may not have the energy for both. By limiting your obligations you will be able to lower the stress in your life. Some people also find meditation or yoga to be helpful in reducing the stress in their lives. Yoga may not only help you reduce your stress level, but it may also help you feel physically better as well.

Attitude Is Everything

It is believed, by some, that your attitude toward your illness has a lot to do with how well your body responds to treatment and how well you do in the long run. Your attitude may be linked to your immune system and how it responds. This makes sense on a practical level if you think about it. For example, if you have a bad attitude about getting better, you may not be as compliant as you should be. You may not listen to the important things that your doctor is telling you. You may not pay attention to your body's needs. You may not do all the things that you know you are supposed to be doing to get well and keep your body in top form.

"I hated going to the hospital for my treatments. I actually used to cry and sometimes I would even stay at my friend's house so that my parents could not find me when it was time to go," says Julia. "I hated that I had leukemia. I didn't want to take my treatments. I guess I thought I was just going to die anyway so what I did really did not matter.

"Then one of my teachers asked me to talk to her after school one day. She said that she noticed that I wasn't doing my homework anymore and that I wasn't paying much attention in school. She asked me what was going on at home. She already knew that I had leukemia, but she was asking me to tell her about what was going on with me. She was one of my favorite teachers and so I felt pretty comfortable telling her the truth. I'm so glad I did because then she said she had something to tell me.

74

"She said that when she was in high school she had gotten leukemia, too. I could hardly believe it. She looked so healthy and normal. She was alive, standing there alive in front of me. She helped me understand that I really had to take my treatments and do what the doctors told me to do. Also, I had to change my attitude and tell myself that I was going to survive. She also told me that she would help and support me, and we could talk whenever I needed to.

"That one conversation made so much difference to me. It was amazing to see that she was an adult who had survived what I was going through. Her friendship and her support helped me change my attitude. I have been in remission for two years now."

Some people even believe that you have power over the things that happen inside your body. Remember how Kat used to pretend to be on a beach during her radiation treatments? Some people like to meditate and visualize the leukemia cells leaving their body. Inside their minds they visualize themselves having a healthy body. Some people enjoy the relaxation effects of meditation or yoga. It helps them to relax and feel calm during their treatments.

If you are interested in finding out about these types of relaxation techniques, look in the yellow pages of your telephone book or ask your doctor. One thing to keep in mind, however, is that these relaxation techniques and visualizations of good health are not an alternative to the treatments your doctor is prescribing for you. They are a supplement, something to give you an extra boost to help you get through your treatments and illness.

"I just did what my doctors told me I had to do," says Kat. *"My grandma had cancer at the same time as I did and I saw how she handled it. She was so strong. She would just say stuff like, 'Well, the doctor says to do this, so that is what I do. I don't waste my time worrying about what I cannot fix.'*

"She had such a great attitude, so I did what she did. I let the doctors worry about the big stuff and I just did what they said I should do. I tried really hard to have a good attitude and just deal with things very factually, the way I saw my grandma do it. She really inspired me to be strong and get better."

Should I Keep My Illness a Secret?

The fact that you have leukemia is nothing to be ashamed of. You will probably find that it is in your best interest to let people know that you have leukemia. Your teachers, especially, will need to know if you will be missing a lot of school. If you tell them why you are missing school, they will be able to make proper arrangements to help you get your work so that you can keep up with your classmates. If you spend extended periods of time in the hospital, you may be able to get a tutor to help you stay caught up with your classes so that when you get back to school you will not have missed much. Your friends may also prove to be highly valuable allies in your fight against leukemia.

"When I first got sick," says Aidan, seventeen, "I didn't want anyone to come to visit me, but the guys

on my block insisted on coming by. They brought me magazines, movies, homework, and great stories about all the stuff that was going on at school. They were sort of like my lifeline to the outside world. They always told me about things that were coming up, too. You know, like things that they knew I wouldn't want to miss. They encouraged me to look forward to stuff so I would get better and actually get to do the things they were describing. I sometimes wonder if I would have made it without them."

Having an illness like leukemia is nothing to be embarrassed about. It is no one's fault that you are sick, and you have no reason to be ashamed about the fact that you are ill. By sharing information regarding your illness with your friends, you will help them understand what you are going through. This in turn will guide them in knowing how to help you deal with things.

"I was embarrassed when I started to lose my hair from chemo," says Eliot, now nineteen. "I decided to shave my head because I thought it would look better than having only a little bit of hair. I went to school with a hat on the first day, but the kids in my class wanted to see what I looked like bald, so I took it off. I couldn't believe what happened the next day. Every single guy in my class came back to school with his head shaved. It was incredible. It was the most amazing and touching show of support I could ever have imagined."

Living with Leukemia

This is a very stressful time for you. You may have to miss school and other activities that are important to you. You may often feel sick. You may lose your hair. Although these things can all cause you to get upset, continuing to see your friends, play sports, and go to school will help you keep high hopes. Do these things as much as your illness allows you to, but accept your limits. Taking care of your body has to come first. When you are feeling well, go ahead and do all of your regular activities, but when you are not feeling well, set a goal in your mind that will remind you how soon you will be well enough to do them again. Planning for your future while you are sick will provide you with reasons to get well. This is an important part of your recovery.

"When I first found out that I had leukemia I got mad and thought for sure that I was going to die," says Ryan, eighteen. "I didn't want to go to school anymore, and I quit the football team. I just didn't see the point in doing anything anymore. But then I found out something very interesting about my doctor that changed the way I felt about everything. Dr. Grant had leukemia when he was a teenager, just like me. He started college while he was still sick. He got better and went on

to medical school. When I met him he was not only still fine, he was my inspiration."

Your Family

Although you are the one who has leukemia, your family may also be experiencing emotional changes, too. It might do you some good to try to be sensitive to their feelings. They may be afraid of losing you. They may feel guilty that they are healthy and enjoying their regular activities while you are sick and fighting to get well.

Your mom and dad, for example, may feel confused, angry, or scared because they love you so much and they are so afraid of what might happen if you do not get better. They may be wondering why you got sick and if there was anything they could have done to prevent it. They may also feel burdened by the time they have to take off from work and the fact that your care may be very expensive. You should try to understand this stress, but do not let it stress you. Your mom and dad are there to take care of you. It is their job.

If you have brothers and sisters, they may not understand what is happening to you or why you are getting so much attention. They may also be frightened by the thought that if you got sick they could, too. Younger brothers and sisters may think it was their fault that you got sick because they said or did something they were not supposed to do.

"I remember thinking that Emily got leukemia because I had been mean to her," says Bobby, now twelve. "She was always trying to play with my stuff *and one day I told her I wished she would go away and never come back. A couple of weeks later she got sick. I know now that Emily's getting sick was not my fault, but at the time I felt like a really horrible brother."*

Letting your family members in on what is happening to you will help them to be less frightened. Also, if you or your family members have questions, the people who have the best answers are your nurses and doctors. Ask them all the questions you feel the need to have answered. These health care professionals not only know the concrete facts about leukemia, they also understand what you and your family are going through emotionally.

"I used to write in my journal about what happened when I was at the hospital getting chemo," says Kim, seventeen. "I also wrote about how having leukemia made me feel. On Sunday nights after my family had dinner, I would bring out my journal and my sister and brother would take turns reading what I had written about during the past week. Then my mom and dad would read it. I think it helped everyone deal with the situation better, knowing exactly what I was going through."

A Friend Like Me

"When I first got sick with leukemia, I felt really alone," says Janelle, seventeen. "I was sure that I was the only teenager in the world to get a disease. I didn't think any of my friends would understand

what I was going through because they were not sick themselves. But the first time I had to go into the hospital I met some other people who had leukemia. There was Bella, a little girl who was only six, Anthony, who was fifteen, and Deirdre, who was my age. Deirdre and I spent a lot of time talking. We had so much in common. It made me feel really normal to have a friend who was going through the same things I was going through."

Ask around at your hospital or your cancer clinic to find out if there are other teens who have leukemia and other types of cancer.

If you are not the person who has leukemia, but you are reading this book because someone you know has leukemia, it may be hard to recognize that your friend or sibling with leukemia may feel uncomfortable around you simply because you do not have leukemia. You are no longer the same. This can be difficult for the person who has leukemia to deal with.

"My best friend, Angela, got sick with leukemia last year," says Morgan, sixteen. "I tried really hard to be supportive and be there for her, but the more I tried to help her out the more she pushed me away. We talked and she said that she didn't want me to help her. She didn't want me to act differently toward her because she was sick. She told me just to treat her the way I always had. So I went back to talking about guys in our class, movies, books, and school, instead of asking her how she felt all the time. Angela was a lot happier then, and our friend-

ship went back to being normal. Angela just wanted to be treated the same as usual."

Most people, even when they are sick, just want you to treat them the way you have always treated them. Keeping things as normal as possible is important. Of course, there will be exceptions to this, but you will simply have to assess the situation and maybe even talk it out with your friend who is sick. The best advice is that if you are not sure how your friend or sibling wants to be treated, just ask him or her.

Camps

"The coolest thing that happened when I had leukemia was that I got to go away to overnight camp where all the kids had leukemia," says Michelle, twelve. "All the kids were just like me. It was great. I was bald then, and I was really self-conscious about it. But half the children at camp were bald, and after a day I forgot that being bald was unusual."

Children who have leukemia and other forms of cancer often have the opportunity, if their health permits them, to go to overnight camps designed especially for cancer patients. You do all the things you would do at any other overnight camp, such as swimming, crafts, campfires, and sports. The only difference is that there are trained medical personnel on staff at the camp to help out with medicines and treatments that kids who have cancer may need.

The great thing about going to camp is that unlike at

school or in your neighborhood where you might be the only kid who has cancer, at camp you are surrounded by teens and children who understand your battle because they are fighting it, too. You are just like everyone else. You will have the chance to talk to the other kids about what having leukemia is like for them. Most likely, you will make some very special and very terrific friends.

Remission

"I just do what my doctors tell me," says Joy, fifteen. "They know what they're doing, and they will do the best they can to get me well. So I just take things as they come, do what my doctors tell me, and go about things in my life as if I were still healthy. Sometimes I don't feel well and I have to stay home from school. But I try not to let that get me down. I use the time to catch up on my reading if I am feeling up to it, or my grandma comes over and sits with me and tells me stories about her friend who died of leukemia before I was born. Hearing about her makes me even more determined to survive. One day I want to be telling my granddaughter about how I survived leukemia."

What Is Remission?

Remission is the goal, the state of health you will be in when chemo, radiation, or other therapies have destroyed all of the leukemia cells in your body. This means no evidence of cancer or leukemia will show up in your body when you are tested because there will not be identifiable leukemia cells in your body. Normal blood cell production will resume and blood counts will once again be at healthy levels. You will feel good again. Any leftover leukemia cells in your body will not be able to do any harm, as there are not enough of them to interfere with your functioning.

Most cancers are not considered cured until you have been in remission for about five years. Most children who have leukemia will need to go through intense chemotherapy before they reach complete remission. One thing to remember is that any residual leukemia cells left in your body after chemo, even if they are not active at the moment, can still start to grow out of control again. If this happens, your leukemia will return and you will no longer be in remission. This is called a relapse. Not all people relapse after they achieve remission. In fact, the probability that you will reach remission from acute lymphocytic leukemia and that it will last is well over 75 percent now. If 75 percent does not seem like good odds to you, consider the fact that in 1960 the probability of recovery was only about 5 percent.

If you do have a relapse of leukemia, you will have to start chemo again. The next round of chemo will probably involve a different set of drugs than the ones used when you were first diagnosed. Which drugs your doctor uses will depend on several factors—how old you are, how long you were in remission, and what the leukemia cells look like. Another approach to achieving remission a second time is a stem cell transplant or bone marrow transplant, which we talked about in chapter 7.

Staying Well

Children and teens who have acute lymphocytic leukemia usually continue to receive chemo even after they have achieved remission. This is because some residual leukemia cells may continue to hide in the blood and bone marrow, where they will not be detectable. To keep them from becoming active again, you will need to stay on chemo for a while, although you will probably have a different set of drugs after you achieve remission.

This is a very frightening time you are going through. Doctors, researchers, and scientists have worked very hard to develop treatments for different kinds of leukemia, and they are making great progress with some of them. For example, kids with acute lymphocytic leukemia have an 81 percent chance of recovering. Unfortunately, not all types of leukemia are as treatable as this one. People who get acute myelogenous leukemia have a much lower chance of surviving. Sadly, life-threatening illnesses, like leukemia, are a battle that some people do not survive.

Just for Teens

This chapter is for the teens in the family who do not have leukemia. Earlier, there was a discussion about how the person who has leukemia might treat his or her family while he or she is sick. If you are living in a house where someone has leukemia, you may be having some feelings of your own about all of this. Let us address some of these feelings and emotions that you may be going through. After all, this can be a very scary time for you, too.

You know that your sister or brother probably felt afraid, worried, even angry when she or he found out about having leukemia. But how did you feel? Did anyone talk to you about your feelings? Did anyone explain leukemia to you? Well, hopefully you have found out the facts you wanted to know about leukemia by reading this book. In case no one has addressed your feelings about having a brother or sister who has leukemia, this chapter is just for you.

Emotional Times

Leukemia is a serious disease. It is very frightening to think that if your brother or sister does not get proper treatment, he or she could die. Watching your sister or brother get sick and struggle to get better will be very hard for you. It is understandable that you and your family are pretty worried right now, and you may be experiencing a lot of emotions that you have never felt before.

"When my family first found out that Jamica was sick, my brother, Eric, and I felt totally ignored," says Troy, eleven. "I was really scared that Jamica would die, but I could not even ask my mom and dad about it because they were so busy taking care of her. Eric and I felt left out, scared, worried, and angry all at the same time."

The combination of emotions that Troy and Eric were feeling is very normal. When one of the children in the family is sick for a long period of time, things can get pretty hectic around your house, especially at first. Your mom and dad may have to spend a lot of time at the hospital with your brother or sister. Remember that your mom and dad are as worried and frightened as you are, and so they both want to be there with your sibling who is sick. One of your parents may even stay overnight at the hospital for the duration of the time your sibling has to stay in the hospital. It can be rough having just one parent at home when you are used to having both your mom and dad around.

"My mom stayed at the hospital with Tyler, and my dad stayed home with Valerie and me," says Kathy, eighteen. "But he was hardly home either. As soon as he would come home from work he changed his clothes, asked us if we had done our homework, and then he was back out the door to go visit my mom and Tyler at the hospital. It was really hard on Valerie

and me. We were alone a lot. Tyler was sick, but we needed our mom and dad, too. Luckily, as Tyler got better, my dad relaxed a bit and sometimes he didn't go to the hospital after work and instead he would take Valerie and me to the movies or something special like that. When Tyler came home, things got a lot more normal again."

Your sibling who has leukemia may have to go in and out of the hospital or to the clinic for treatments fairly often. For a while you may just have to get used to this, but it will not be forever. Some kids stay with other family members, friends, or neighbors while their sibling is in the hospital. This can add to your stress because for a time you have to get used to living with different people and without all of your belongings and familiar surroundings.

Being Concerned and Worried

Your sister or brother is going through a really rough time because fighting cancer is not easy. The medicines that are being used to fight off the leukemia are hard on the healthy cells in your sibling's body, too. This is why your sibling may feel lousy, lose his or her hair, lose or gain weight, and not look like his or her usual self.

Are you worrying about your sick sibling a lot? This is okay. It is hard to watch someone you love go through these things. You may even feel strange about doing your normal activities when you know your brother or sister is too sick to do much more than lie on the sofa and watch television.

"I used to worry that Jamica would be jealous or upset with me because I was still playing basketball after school while she was at home sick," says Troy. "I asked her how she felt and she said she was glad that I was still doing all of my regular stuff. She said it made things seem more normal around the house.

"When I would come home from a game or a practice, Jamica asked me lots of questions about things that she missed. She said she liked to hear about the things that I was doing and she also said it gave her something to think about doing when she got well. Now that she is better, Jamica plays basketball too."

Sadness and Guilt

Some teens cry when they find out that their brother or sister has leukemia. This is a perfectly normal reaction. Sadness is a very normal emotion to have when someone you love is sick. When your brother or sister starts to feel better, you will also start to feel better.

Why is your sister or brother sick while you are still healthy? There is no answer for that question. Even so, you may still experience some feelings of guilt because you are healthy and you can still do everything that you have always done, while your sibling is getting treatments, losing his or her hair, and fighting to get better.

You may also be wondering if something you did caused your sibling to get leukemia. However, you are not responsible for your sibling's illness. Nothing you said, did, or thought caused your brother or sister to get leukemia. Even if you were really mad at him or her, the fact that your sibling got sick and you did not is really just a matter of chance. It is no more your fault that your sibling is sick than it is his or her fault. The fact that your sister or brother has leukemia is nobody's fault.

Jealousy

There is no doubt that your sick sibling is getting quite a bit of extra attention these days. Although on the surface you probably understand why this is happening, deep down you may still be feeling some jealousy over this extra attention. Your sibling may be receiving gifts, phone calls, flowers, and cards. You may be feeling neglected because your mom and dad are focusing so much time and energy on your sibling. You may feel left out, which may lead you to having feelings of jealousy toward your sibling.

It is normal to feel jealous. Actually, although your sibling may be sick, he or she is getting to do some things that you may wish you could do, like staying home from school, getting presents and attention, and having extra time with your mom and dad. If you are afraid that people are treating your sick sibling differently because they love him or her better, do not worry. How much you and your brothers and sisters are loved has nothing to do with who has leukemia and who is healthy. Your mom and dad and other relatives love you as much as they always have, just as you still love them the same as you did before your sibling got sick. It is important to remember that these special things are being done to help your brother or sister get better. It is okay to be upset about all of this. After all, you are under stress as well. Your frustration over everything being about your brother or sister is really normal. Do not forget that if you were the one who was sick, you would be getting all the attention.

Loneliness

Your brother or sister is at the hospital, and your mom and dad are at the hospital, too. You are left at home missing everyone. It is very normal if you miss your sibling, your mom and dad, and the way things used to be before leukemia became part of your family.

While your brother or sister and one or both of your parents are at the hospital, there are a few things that you can do to feel less lonely. Write letters and make cards to send to your sibling at the hospital. Talk with them on the phone for a few minutes every day. Spend some extra time with your friends or with relatives whom you really like. Visit your sibling at the hospital if you can.

Then, when your brother or sister and your parents are all home again, ask for a bit of special time just for you. Perhaps your mom will take you shopping one afternoon, or your dad will take you out for lunch. You may even want to spend some one-on-one time with your sibling who has leukemia. It is important for the two of you to support each other and maintain a healthy relationship while all of this is going on. If your sibling does not feel well enough to go out, you can certainly do what Sara and Victor used to do when Victor was sick.

"I made this really big sign that said, 'Sara and Victor Time, Do Not Disturb' and I would hang it on Victor's bedroom door when we felt like we hadn't

had much time together lately. Usually I would bring up a bunch of junk food, like all of our favorite cookies and chips and sometimes ice cream. We would just hang out in there for hours watching television or playing cards. Sometimes we would read magazines together and other times we wrote stories. It was nice to spend time together, just the two of us.

"Now that Victor is better, we still get together for 'Sara and Victor Time.' But now we go out and ride our bikes, go to the movies, or walk to the mall or the beach."

Confusion

Why is my brother or sister sick? How long will he or she be sick? What will he or she have to go through to try to get well? Will it hurt? Will anything ever be the same again? This is a very confusing time for you and everyone in your family. You may notice that different members of your family do not react to things the same way that they used to. For example, perhaps your father no longer seems concerned over whether or not you finish your dinner before you get dessert, or maybe your mom yells at you more than she used to over little things that would not have bothered her in the past.

Perhaps you react to things differently, too. Maybe homework has become overwhelming or you do not feel like keeping your room clean anymore. You may not feel like talking to your friends right now. Even your dog may be acting nervous and hyper. Everyone is confused. Everyone is dealing with their own feelings and emotions. None of you knows how all of this is going to turn out. All of you hope for the best, but you probably all fear the worst, even if you are afraid to say so out loud. You may also be confused about the things that are happening when your brother or sister goes into the hospital.

Ask questions if you feel you need to understand something better. Another thing you can do is ask to go to the hospital and see for yourself all the things that your brother or sister is going through. Meet the nurses and doctors who are taking care of your sister or brother. See the hospital, the rooms, and the clinic where your sibling is going to be spending his or her time. Check out the machines that deliver your brother's or sister's medicines and treatments. Once you have had a chance to get familiar with all of these things, you will have less confusion over what is going on.

Fear

What are you afraid of? You may be afraid that your brother or sister is going to die. You may be afraid of what will happen to the rest of your family if your brother or sister does not get well. You may be afraid that you are going to have to watch your sibling getting worse, throwing up, losing hair, and looking sick. You may fear death itself, as all of a sudden it has become a very real possibility in your family. You may fear the pain your sibling might have to endure.

Remember that any feeling you have about everything that is going on right now is very real and completely valid. Do not feel guilty about whatever feelings you have. Trying to pretend that you are not having an emotional reaction to the fact that your sister or brother has

93

leukemia will not help you at all. Identifying and facing your feelings will help you a great deal.

What If I Don't Feel Bad at All?

For most people, a diagnosis of a serious illness such as leukemia can bring out strong feelings. However, some people have a lot of confidence in the new treatments that are available today. Instead of worrying about things over which they have little or no control, they simply go about their usual activities and trust that the doctors will do all they can to help their brother or sister get well.

"I really didn't worry all that much when I found out that my sister Jaime had leukemia," says Hudson, seventeen. "I mean, I knew it was a serious disease, but I also knew that there was a pretty good chance that she would get better. I had known a kid at school whose brother had leukemia a few years before. He was fine, so I just figured Jaime would get treatments and eventually she would be fine, too. I just did not get upset and worry about things that were pretty much out of our control."

It is okay not to feel upset over your brother's or sister's leukemia. Everyone feels their own way. Everyone handles stressful, serious, or difficult situations in their own way. How you choose to deal with your sibling's leukemia is personal to you. No one can tell you that you should be upset or that you should not worry. Your instincts and your own experiences will dictate how you feel, and however you feel is okay.

Some Ways to Cope with Your Feelings

This book is about coping with leukemia, whether it is your leukemia or leukemia suffered by someone you love. Children and teens who have leukemia or other life-threatening illnesses, and those people who are close to them, have to find special ways of coping within their unique situations.

Everyone has his or her own way of coping when things get tough. The following is a list of suggestions that may help you cope with leukemia. You may choose to try all of the suggestions or maybe just one or two that sound like the best options for you. Remember that everyone copes with things differently and the way you choose to cope may be entirely different from the way someone else chooses to cope.

- Keep a journal. Write about your feelings, thoughts, fears, hopes, and questions. Write about whatever comes to your mind as often as you feel like writing. Your journal may be private or you may choose to share it with others.

- Talk about it. Talk about your feelings with your family. Find out how everyone else is feeling and how they are dealing with and coping with this change in your family's life.

- Ask questions. Ask nurses and doctors to explain things to you. If you or your loved one is about to have a certain procedure done, ask for the details or a step-by-step explanation of what is going to be happening.

⮑ Face your feelings. If you are afraid, feel afraid. If you are angry, feel your anger. Whatever emotion or emotions you are experiencing, really take time to feel them. Holding your feelings inside and not acknowledging them will only make you feel worse in the long run.

⮑ Get support. Join a support group for teens who have leukemia or for siblings of children and teens who have leukemia. Talking to people who are going through the same things that you are going through can be enormously helpful.

Learning All You Can

Learning about leukemia and understanding what is going on inside the body will help make things easier to cope with. Find books that tell you the facts, but also look for books that tell stories of teens who have dealt with leukemia. Search the Internet for information. A list of resources can be found at the end of this book.

Above all else, know that the doctors and the health care team are doing everything in their power to help you or your loved one get well. Stay strong. Fight hard. Take each day as it comes and face the challenges in front of you. People who have leukemia have a very good chance of going into remission. Hopefully, once remission is achieved, you or your loved one will remain healthy for a very long time. Do not give up. You never know when someone will come along with a new treatment or even a cure for leukemia. The future is bright. Make the future yours.

Glossary

acute   Sudden onset, develops quickly.

acute lymphocytic leukemia (ALL)   Type of leukemia that affects both children and adults; accounts for just over half of all cases of childhood leukemia.

acute myelogenous leukemia (AML)   Leukemia that affects both children and adults; accounts for just under half of all cases of childhood leukemia.

anemia   A condition that occurs when a person's body does not have enough red blood cells.

antibodies   Proteins produced by the body in response to contact with an antigen, also has the ability to neutralize or react with the antigen.

basophils   The rarest of all white blood cells.

B cells   Cells that are responsible for making antibodies to kill off foreign substances that find their way into your body.

benign   The opposite of malignant, not cancerous.

bone marrow   A soft and spongy substance found on the inside of bones. It is made of cells that form blood, fat cells, and the tissues that help the blood cells grow.

carcinogens   Things that cause cancer.

chronic lymphocytic leukemia (CLL)   Leukemia that affects adults only; almost twice as common as chronic myelogenous leukemia.

chronic myelogenous leukemia (CML)   Leukemia that is very
   rare for children, affecting mostly adults; about half as common as chronic lymphocytic leukemia.
differentiation   The process by which all of the stem cells
   grow up and turn into the different types of cells that make
   up your blood.
enzyme   The protein in the cells that proofreads the DNA and
   corrects an error before it can cause any serious damage.
eosinophils   White blood cells that help fight off parasites
   and bad bacteria; also respond to allergic reactions.
erythrocytes   Another name for red blood cells.
genes   The parts of DNA that contain the actual instructions
   that tell your body's cells when to grow and divide normally.
graft   When new bone marrow merges with your system and
   starts to make new, healthy blood cells.
granulocytes   One of the two main types of white blood
   cells that play very specific roles in protecting your body
   from infection.
immunotherapy   A possible leukemia treatment of the future
   in which the body's natural defenses are built up and made
   stronger so that they can do the work of preventing or
   killing leukemia cells.
leukocytes   Another name for white blood cells.
lymphatic system   A complex system in the body that
   resembles the veins but carries a substance other than blood.
lymphocytes   One of the two main types of white blood
   cells that play very specific roles in protecting your body
   from infection.
lymphocytic   One of the types of cells that starts leukemia.
malignancy   Another word for cancer.
metastasis   When cancer cells travel from an original site to
   new areas of the body and keep growing there.
monocytes   White blood cells that have special enzymes that
   kill off bad bacteria.

myelogenous Cancer that begins from one of two types of white blood cells, the monocytes or the granulocytes; also called myeloid or myelocytic.

neutrophils The largest group of white blood cells; responsible for action when bad bacteria gets into the body.

oncogenes Specific genes responsible for cell division.

oncologist Cancer doctor.

pathologist Doctor who specializes in analyzing body tissues.

pediatric oncologist A children's cancer doctor.

platelets Pieces that have broken off from some of the bone marrow cells that help form blood clots; also known as thrombocytes.

prognosis How well you do with treatment.

radiation oncologist Doctor who specializes in using radiation to treat cancer.

radiation therapy A way of treating cancer by using penetrating beams of high-energy waves or streams of particles.

radioimmunotherapy Injection of antibodies with attached isotopes that emit radiation into a leukemia patient's body; type of immunotherapy.

red blood cells Blood cells that carry oxygen away from the lungs and out to all of the other tissues in the body; also known as erythrocytes.

rejection When your body does not accept the new or transplanted bone marrow the way it should.

remission State of health you will be in after chemo, radiation, or other medicines or therapies have destroyed all of the leukemia cells in your body.

stem cells Young blood cells.

T cells Cells that attack cancer cells, infected cells, and foreign bodies.

translocation When DNA from one chromosome attaches itself to the wrong chromosome after division.

tumor   A group of cancer cells that bunch together to form a mass or a lump.

tumor suppressor genes   Genes responsible for slowing down cell growth and division and making sure that cells die off when they are supposed to.

white blood cells   Blood cells that help the body defend itself against infections; also called leukocytes.

Where to Go for Help

American Cancer Society
1599 Clifton Road NE
Atlanta, GA 30329
(800) ACS-2345
Web site: http://www.cancer.org

Leukemia & Lymphoma Society of America
475 Park Avenue South, 21st Floor
New York, NY 10016
(800) 955-4572
Web site: http://www.leukemia.org

National Bone Marrow Donor Program
3433 Broadway Street NE, Suite 500
Minneapolis, MN 55413
(800) 654-1247
Web site: http://www.marrow.org

National Children's Leukemia Foundation
172 Madison Avenue
New York, NY 10016
(800) GIVE HOPE (448-3467)
Web site: http://www.leukemiafoundation.org

Pall Corporation
2200 Northern Boulevard
East Hills, NY 11548
(516) 484-5400
Web site: http://www.bloodtransfusion.com

For Further Reading

Jaffe, Hirshel, James Rudin, and Marsha Rudin. *Why Me? Why Anyone?* Northvale, NJ: Jason Aronson Publisher, 1994.

Keene, Nancy. *Childhood Leukemia: A Guide for Families, Friends & Caregivers.* Cambridge, MA: O'Reilly & Associates, Incorporated, 1999.

Krumme, Cynthia. *Having Leukemia Isn't So Bad: Of Course It Wouldn't Be My First Choice.* Winchester, MA: Sargasso Enterprises, 1993.

Laszlo, John. *The Cure of Childhood Leukemia: In the Age of Miracles.* Piscataway, NJ: Rutgers University Press, 1996.

Lilleyman, John S. *Childhood Leukemia: The Facts* (The Facts Series). New York: Oxford University Press, 1994.

Siegel, Dorothy S., and David E. Newton. *Leukemia.* Danbury, CT: Franklin Watts Incorporated, 1994.

Westcott, Patsy. *Living with Leukemia* (Living with Series). Chatham, NJ: Raintree Steck-Vaughn, 1999.

Index

A

acute lymphocytic leukemia
(ALL), 15, 22–23, 41,
84, 85
acute myelogenous leukemia
(AML), 14, 18, 21, 22,
23–24, 28, 29, 36, 85
anemia, 8, 13, 15–16, 43
appetite, loss of, 13, 14, 41,
71–72

B

balance problem, 13, 14
B cells, 10, 59
blast cells, 19, 23
blood, 3, 4, 6, 7–8, 10, 23,
43, 58, 60, 61, 64, 65,
84, 85
transfusions, 43–44
blood cells
red, 3, 4, 7, 8, 14, 15, 18,
23, 43, 58
white, 3, 4, 6, 7, 8, 9, 10,
14, 19, 21, 23, 28, 58,
62, 64
bone marrow, 3, 6, 7, 8, 9, 14,
19, 22, 23, 30, 41, 44,
58, 59, 60, 64, 65, 85

donor, 60–68
donor drive, 62
extracting, 19, 67–68
National Marrow Donor
Program, 61–68
siblings and parents as,
60–61, 63
bone marrow transplant (BMT),
24, 58–68, 69, 84
rejection, 65
breath, shortness of, 8, 13,
15, 16
bruising, 4, 9, 13, 18

C

camps, 82–83
cancer, 3, 4–5, 21, 29, 30,
32–33, 41, 44, 45,
50–52, 53, 82, 83–84
cures for, 5–6
new drugs for, 47–49
carcinogens, 32, 34
catheter, indwelling, 46
chemical spills, 32, 35, 36
chemotherapy, 24, 36, 37,
40–49, 51, 52, 64, 66
83–84, 85
how it works, 44–45

side effects of, 41–44,
47, 51, 88
where given, 45–46
Chernobyl accident, 32
chromosomes, 24, 31, 33
chronic lymphocytic
leukemia, 22
chronic myelogenous
leukemia (CML), 22

D

DNA, 23, 30, 31, 32, 33
translocation of, 31
doctor, seeing your, 16,
18–19, 27, 36, 38,
44, 47, 48, 51, 56,
57, 64, 66, 70, 72,
75, 80, 85, 94, 96
Down's syndrome, 23–24,
29, 33–34
drug trials, 48–49

E

eating right, 71–72
exercise, 70–71

F

fatigue/weakness, 4, 8, 12,
14, 16, 41, 69, 70,
72, 88
Federal Drug Administration
(FDA), 48

G

graft, 65
gum bleeds, 9, 13, 14

H

hair loss, 40, 41, 43, 78, 88,
89, 93
hospital, going to, 36–39,
45–46, 53, 64, 69,
76, 88, 91, 93
Human Leukocyte Antigen
(HLA) type, 61–62,
63, 66

I

immune system, 11, 35, 37,
65, 73, 74
immunotherapy, 49
infection, 3, 7, 9, 10, 11,
18, 23, 37, 43, 44,
47, 65
iron in diet, 8, 16, 71

L

leukemia
adults and, 4, 22, 23, 24,
29, 35
attitude and, 74–75
children/teens and, 4,
19, 21, 22, 23, 24,
28, 29, 35, 37, 41,
69, 81–83, 85, 95
chronic, 21, 22, 29
diagnosis of, 1, 2, 12,
14, 17–21, 25–26,
38, 69
environment and, 4,
32–33, 34, 36
family and, 1, 26, 37 63,
73, 79–80, 86–96

feelings about, 2, 25, 26,
	27 78, 79, 80, 85,
	86–96
fighting it, 2, 26, 27, 49,
	71, 72, 88, 89, 96
friends and, 1, 26, 72,
	76, 77, 78, 81–83
heredity and, 4, 23, 30,
	34, 35, 36
learning about, 1, 2, 7,
	11, 27, 96
no one's fault, 35, 36,
	77, 89–90
prevent, no way to, 35
remission of, 83–84,
	85, 96
school and, 69, 70, 71,
	72, 73, 76, 78
statistics about, 28, 29
symptoms of, 1, 3, 4, 9,
	12–14, 16, 18, 20, 69
treatment for, 1, 16, 24,
	26, 27, 28, 36, 38,
	39, 40, 51, 58, 69,
	75, 82, 85, 96
what it is, 3–4, 5–6, 9,
	10, 28, 35, 36
when a loved one has it,
	86–96
lymphatic system, 7, 8, 10–11
lymph nodes, 6, 10, 11, 14 18
lymphoma, 35

M
malignancy, 5
metastasis, 5

N
nosebleeds, 9, 13
nurses, 27, 38, 39, 44, 57,
	80

O
oncogenes, 30, 31

P
patient rights, 27, 38–39
plasma, 7, 58, 59
platelets, 3, 4, 7, 8–9, 14,
	18, 23, 43, 58, 64
protective isolation, 64

R
radiation, exposure to, 23,
	32–33, 35, 36
radiation therapy, 24, 36,
	37, 41, 50–57, 66,
	75, 83
	combination therapy,
		51, 64
	facts about, 52–53
	how given, 53–55
	how it works, 50–51,
		54–56
	side effects of, 51, 52
	tips about, 56–57
recovery, 64, 65, 85
relapse, 65, 84
relaxation techniques,
	73, 75

S
skin, pale, 13, 16

sleep, 72–73
stem cells, 8, 59, 60, 84
stress, 70, 73, 79, 88, 90
superior vena cava, 15
surgery, 41, 51
SVC syndrome, 15

T
T cells, 10, 15, 35, 59
tumors, 4–5, 6, 24, 51–52
    chloroma, 18, 24

tumor suppressor genes,
    30

V
viruses, 4, 9, 34–35
vomiting, 13, 14, 40,
    41–42, 93

W
weight loss/gain, 12, 14,
    72, 88